paper dollhouse

A Memoir

DR. LISA M. MASTERSON

Guilford, Connecticut
An imprint of Globe Pequot Press

skirt!® is an attitude . . . spirited, independent, outspoken, serious, playful and irreverent, sometimes controversial, always passionate.

Text design: Sheryl P. Kober
Layout: Joanna Beyer

Library of Congress Cataloging-in-Publication Data is available on file.

ISBN 978-1-59921-998-1

Printed in the United States of America
10 9 8 7 6 5 4 3 2 1

This book is dedicated to my mother, La V'onne,
my son, Daniel, and my husband, Steve,
the three pillars of my life.

Contents

Introduction

It's just a few minutes until our call to the stage for the taping of another episode of *The Doctors*, and on this day I'm sitting backstage with my briefing book closed in my lap, mulling over the topic I'll be discussing with one of our cohosts, Dr. Travis Stork. I've talked about breast cancer thousands of times with my patients, but I've rarely spoken in public about my mom's encounter with the disease, and thinking about it brings a surge of emotion. I was in medical school when my mom was diagnosed, and I was a doctor in training at USC when I lost her. Mom was my whole life, and I feel her beside me as I steady myself to tell her story. I know she'd be proud to know that she's helping me remind thousands of women to take the steps that can save their lives.

My mom was my best friend and biggest supporter, and as I'll say on the show, I owe everything to her unflagging belief in me. It was the one thing I had in abundance growing up in a crazy childhood that seems almost impossibly far from here.

My mother and I sit at the kitchen table, the white Formica spread with my schoolwork and a jumble of mail. I have a good head for numbers, and I may be the only kid in my fourth-grade class who likes word problems. My mom throws one at me.

"Phone bill," she says, opening an envelope and frowning at what she sees. "Okay, Leese. What'll we do with this one?"

Here's the long version of the problem: A single mom and her daughter live in Seattle. The mom's government job pays enough to cover all the bills except tuition for the daughter's exclusive private school. Subtract the pricey education and the numbers all line up.

But that would mean erasing the mom's vision for the daughter, which involves strapping her girl to a rocket and sending her flying past the barriers that are still stacked in front of a black child in the 1970s. So: dream or duty? What do you do when the phone bill comes due?

"No signature," I say. It'll take a while for the phone company to deal with our "honest mistake" when they get the unsigned check. We're behind, and we don't want them to shut us off again. But maybe this will buy us some time. Sometimes it does.

For other bills, at times like now when we're strapped, we've got other answers. There's "wrong date," "send to the wrong address," "mix up the checks"—by putting, say, a check for the phone company in the utility-bill envelope. At age nine I know them all well. This is what we do; it binds us together. It boosts me up and sends me to class with the rich kids.

I often tell people that my mother was the most important person in my life. They look at me, look at my résumé. It's a testament to her influence. I went to prep schools, a Seven Sisters college, med school. I have a beautiful son, a private medical practice, even a job that gives me the opportunity to reach tens of thousands of people with positive messages about living a healthy life and saving the lives of women and children. Because of my mom I believed I could do anything—things like starting a charity that helps fund clinics in Africa and India—and I got the running start that so often comes only with wealth. My life has been sweet and blessed. The years I had with my mom—she died when I was twenty-seven—were filled with our devotion to each other. There were also those nights at the kitchen table, "paying bills" and concocting solutions for keeping our struggling family of two afloat.

Jungians call the push-pull between a person's contradictions the tension of opposites. Malcolm X had another phrase that applies: "by any means necessary." And my mother, La V'onne Smith? She was rhetoric-free and focused solely on pushing open doors in my life, some inner, some outer. She wanted to expand the world's notions—and my own—of what I could be. I'd have to say she succeeded. Because my mom, a smart black woman from Louisiana, went north for a new life, I know what it's like to start from scratch far from home with nothing but your wits to sustain you. I know, too, how often people look at one another and see only what they want to see—or believe that what's in front of them now is an unchangeable reality. I learned early about façades and surfaces and conventional wisdom and the possibilities they hide.

Those lessons were hard won, and sometimes painful, but they have served me in ways you wouldn't expect as I've worked to harness them for the good. When I was a medical student, I heard a statistic that shook me to my core: Every minute a woman in the developing world dies from pregnancy-related causes that are mostly preventable or treatable. And every thirty seconds a child dies as a result of its mother's death. It was hard to bear the thought of this enormous, seemingly intractable chain of loss. I wondered how my mother might respond to those staggering facts. "Throw up your hands" wasn't in her vocabulary. "A step at a time" is what I heard. Though I was just one person, I started to look for ideas and money and ways to begin to shift the odds for some of those women and children.

That's how it happens that in a rural area of northern Kenya where women once walked twenty miles or more to give birth to a baby there is now a small clinic that has saved hundreds of lives. The driving impulse behind that small change for good was a mother's belief—my mother's belief—in her child and the world.

I'm still at work on finding ways to help babies and pregnant women and still facing down the challenges that come with being a human who needs to be Wonder Woman sometimes to get through the day. When I'm alone with my disappointments, or stuck and wondering just what my next step could be, my mother is still the voice in my ear laughing at the naysayers and saying, "We'll find a way."

This is the story of the big love that came from a most unconventional woman. It's messy, and sometimes dark, the way love always is. But it set some amazing futures in motion, and they're part of her story, too. This book and all I've ever accomplished are dedicated to her.

ONE

You and Me against the World

One thing I've always known about my mother: She had enough warmth and fire to melt whatever came between her and a goal that had taken root in her mind. Divorced and solely responsible for me after just a few years of marriage, she used what women have always called on when resources fall short of needs: charm, grit, and ingenuity. She could hatch a plan and charm the pants off anyone to get it going.

When I was three, Mom packed up her well-used car, put me in the front seat next to her, and pointed us away from Haynesville, Louisiana, where her people had lived for generations. The car rode low with the weight of our boxes and bags, and there was no room—in any sense—for my father. He was an English professor and jazz musician—a sax player—and he hadn't taken it well when Mom announced that she didn't need his permission or approval to apply for a job teaching English at the University of Washington in Seattle.

"Where in the hell is that?" is what he probably said, "and what kind of reception does a woman like you think she's going to get that far north? You have got to be out of your mind!"

Whatever argument he mustered, it didn't slow her in the least. When she got word that the job was hers, she steeled herself, grabbed me, and never looked back. My grandmother and the extended family gathered around the car to see us off, shaking their heads but knowing there was no stopping La V'onne Smith. She'd sprinted off to college at sixteen, graduated at nineteen, and chafed against the life that was available to a young black woman in the still-segregated South.

"Mama, I'll call you," she yelled out the window. I watched our old house disappear. We were headed for a whole new life, and I knew that was a good thing.

A long twenty-four hundred miles later, we limped into a gas station, tired, dusty, and down to our last few dollars. The plan for this move hadn't fully taken into account how much gas and rooms on the road would cost, much less what we'd do when we got to the other end. But here we were. It was time to cope.

"You stay in the car now," Mom said as she climbed out, one long, slim leg announcing our arrival and the rest of her curves providing the fanfare. She was always turning heads, and today was no exception. Though there was no question what side of the color line we belonged on in Haynesville, here, with her golden skin; freckles; soft, full lips; and "very keen" nose, as she liked to describe it, she was hard to categorize. "Exotic" seemed to sum her up in the minds of a lot of the people we met. It didn't matter much: By instinct and habit we'd found our way to the city's black neighborhood.

Mom didn't have a Southern accent, but she did have a practiced allure, and today she turned it on. We were country damsels in distress. She flashed her sparkling brown eyes at the station owner, gestured to the license plates on the car, and began to tell our travelers' story. The engine sizzled and dripped.

"You come on out and say hello to Uncle Tom," she called to me after a couple of minutes. Things had come to a standstill at the shop as the mechanics gathered around.

"This little lady looks like she could use a nice cold soda," said the station owner, handing me a coin. I dropped it into the slot of the machine in front of the office, and when a bottle of Grape Crush rolled down the chute of the cooler, he pulled it out and popped off the cap with a grease-stained rag before handing it to me. A little more chatting and laughing and "Uncle Tom" had offered us a place to sleep—he had an empty room in his house, not far from the garage. We unpacked in his spare bedroom as if we were long-lost relatives and with smiles and good Southern cooking, Mom kept us in Uncle Tom's good graces long enough to hustle up the money for a deposit on a place of our own.

I wouldn't be surprised if that deposit was another gift from Tom. He was a gentle, hopeful man with muddy-water eyes that smiled back appreciatively at my mom and me. He kept me filled with grape soda and turned on the sprinkler in the backyard so I could run through it. His mechanics kept an eye on me while Mom was learning the ropes at the university and looking for our next home. "Gimme Shelter" blared from the station's tinny radio during those first weeks. We'd gotten lucky—we'd found it.

Our new life would hinge on luck and kindness and the sort of gullible generosity that people tend to show to a beautiful young woman with a bright little girl. In Mom's view we were worthy of—even entitled to—any good fortune we could make for ourselves. We were trailblazers, escaping the "blacks only" schools and doctors' offices that lingered in Haynesville and setting out on our own. Mom was a lifelong student of literature, the daughter of an English teacher, a university graduate descended from slaves. And within a year of our arrival in Seattle, she had at least one rapidly evolving plot line in her mind. Its protagonist was me. I would be the female of the family who went to all the best schools, mixing with the children of whatever elite we found. There would be nothing holding me back, no excuses, no compromises. We'd do whatever we had to so one of the Smith women would finally be free to show how brilliantly she could shine.

I don't remember the first place we lived. I think it was university housing in Sand Point, the span of a town away from the campus. We both commuted from there to her classes, since there were no mechanics to look after me in our new place and no money for a babysitter. What the college had was students, and that gave us makeshift day care. Mom would settle me into her office while she was in class, leaving me to wear myself out swiveling around in her chair or coloring at her desk. I'd fall asleep on her sofa and wake to find one of her students checking on me. Or she'd put me in a chair at the back of a lecture hall and I'd be lulled by the rhythm of her voice, authoritative and graceful, as she talked about Shakespeare or Huck Finn. I loved the way all eyes were on her as she spoke, and the way the college girls would stop by my seat and say hello or ask to see what I was drawing. It was a given that I'd be one of them someday.

If it was unconventional for a lecturer to have a child with her all day, we used the old sales trick of "acknowledge and ignore." We didn't apologize, and I was well behaved enough to fit in as a little adult, or that's what I thought. I sat and watched as my mother graded papers, explored the hallways while she met with students, and learned to find my own way to the restrooms so I didn't have to interrupt her to ask.

When she finally settled on a preschool program for me, I became a stop on her way to and from work, the traditional commuting arrangement of working moms. That lasted until "the incident"—something having to do with a racial comment directed at me by someone at the school. One of the other kids, I think. Mom pulled me out and began looking for an alternative. She sussed out the reputations of the public and private schools in the area, then scraped together the money for the private school that inevitably rose to the top. I'd be responsible for getting there and back on my own.

I missed my grandma, but I was fine without my father. He and my mom had split up before the move, and I knew it was my mother who was "home" to me. Still, Seattle felt strange and new. At Epiphany School, the exclusive Episcopal elementary school that would be my new home base, nothing was familiar. We'd been the rural style of Baptist back in Louisiana, spending Sundays in a white-steepled church where people dressed to the nines for hours of preaching, praying, and calling "Amen" and "Thank you, Jesus!" The women there tried to cool the sultry air with their fans, and children like me dozed against them. Epiphany was wet red brick and rain gray, and the incense, ritual, and grand altar of its chapel were a revelation. God seemed bigger there, and my mother said it was fine to feel that—it didn't matter to God how you prayed as long as you prayed. It was okay, she said, if you got more out of praying one way than another. She was pragmatic, and so was her God.

In her eyes I think it was an advantage that I was one of only two black children in my class. With its sons and daughters of civic leaders and the privileged, Epiphany would be my crystal stair.

Classes were different in a lot of ways than they'd have been in Haynesville. I wore a red plaid jumper, crisp white blouse, and red sweater to school every day and became part of a tradition that I couldn't have found back home. An early head of the school, Robert Spock, was the brother of Benjamin Spock, the noted child expert. Intellectual stimulation, not rote, was the rule, and that suited me. I was one of the talkers, always volunteering an answer or a comment. In the cozy classroom buildings, which were full of nooks, books, and such child-size delights as Venus flytraps, I thrived. I settled into my studies, along with the routine of shuttling from home to school to the university campus to home.

"You're paying how much for that school of hers?"

I could hear my grandmother's voice blasting from the receiver when my mother picked up the phone early on Saturday morning for her mother's weekly call. "You know you can't afford anything like that—on your salary? Have you lost your common sense? You're spoiling that girl."

"Mama, you know how I feel about this," Mom would say, holding the receiver away from her ear. "Tell me about Aunt Geneva."

"You are spoiling that child!" would come the refrain.

My extremely expensive education was a constant point of contention in the family. We were probably paying half my mother's salary in tuition, and I was only in first grade. But she was defiant. If "the best" were available to wealthy children, it would also be available to me. The script was written, and even the finest public school wasn't a potent enough catalyst for its star. Epiphany, she thought, would be a game changer, and she had to have it for me—even on an adjunct professor's salary.

But having it wasn't possible by the usual means. And that's where the sleight of hand—the juggling—came in.

Juggling involved taking a salary of a few hundred dollars a week and making it stretch to include not only the necessities but also the money for that bank-busting tuition check—and all the activities that go with a platinum education: ballet lessons, class trips and activities, camp. I don't know when I first became aware of how she made it work. Maybe it was the second or third time we moved.

Mom would get restless, then turn businesslike. "Leese," she'd say, "get your coat. We're going to check out this ad." She'd have the classifieds of the *Times* or the *Post-Intelligencer*, with ads circled under the "Houses for Rent" or "Duplexes" category. We'd drive to a new neighborhood and find the address, and she'd run the quick calculus of apartment hunters: Price right? Nice place? Anything scary about it? Okay! Let's go inside. Those first couple of times, I went with her to the door, but we learned our lesson fast. She was fair-skinned, but I'd inherited my father's coloring, and there was no question that I was a little black girl, especially with my hair in twin ponytails and tied with ribbons. A smile at my mom could turn into a quick, "Sorry, it's not available" when the person who placed the ad glanced down and saw me. It wasn't the blatant door-slamming we might've met in Haynesville, but we got the message.

"Honey," Mom said, "they're just ignorant. But you'd better stay in the car."

Anyone she fooled into giving us a lease got fooled again when it was time to collect the rent for month three or month four. Our check might "go missing." Or there might be a few earnest promises to pay next week, the week after that for sure, before it became clear that the money wasn't coming at all. A moving van would come, we'd empty one place of our belongings, and we'd set up housekeeping in a brand new spot.

A lot of people can tell you every detail of their childhood homes—the pattern of the wallpaper in their bedroom, the way the shadows tangled through bare branches on a winter night, the way a clock ticked from the hallway into the sound of their dreams. The rooms where they grew up are a part of them. But my homes are a blur, a new one every few months in some years. I was at Epiphany all the way through fourth grade, but I had so many addresses I sometimes had to think before telling someone what part of town I lived in. I knew other people didn't live this way, but I knew exactly why we did: for me. For my education. I was the reason for the flimsy sense of security that dogged us, the new addresses, the distracted look on my mother's face, and the drink in her hand when she sat down at the kitchen table with the bills. And it was my job—my only job—to deserve the gift that was costing us so much. We were a team.

If things had been different—say, if Mom had been a brilliant white woman who was too ambitious for a small, segregated town—it's possible that she never would have had an occasion to drift into the stressful way we lived. Maybe she'd have married a rich man or taken out loans or felt there were enough possibilities for her daughter that there wasn't a need to steal them. Deception was the last thing you'd expect of a woman whose titles would eventually include administrator for the Department of Housing and Urban Development and director of a regional office of the Equal Employment Opportunity Commission. And maybe that's why the juggling was so successful for so long. She wasn't a woman you'd challenge.

Two
Girl Alone

Parenting books will tell you that children need consistency, and in a manner of speaking, I had it. My rock-solid constant was my mother's belief that, left to my own devices, I'd be all right.

I'd been proving that to her all my life. My very first memory is of a commotion in the bathroom when I was two years old. I heard screaming and ran toward it. The room was steamy, and a scalding shower hissed into the tub. My mother struggled in my father's grip as he tried to push her in. Both of them were yelling. His arms were wet. The broom in the corner was bigger than I was, but I grabbed it and jabbed it at him to help my mom pull away. When she did, I ran next door, calling for my great aunt.

That's one of the stories behind our leaving. I think it also helps explain why there was no baby talk between me and my mom. Sometimes it seems as though I was always grown up. She needed me to be.

Our deal was that I would take care of myself when she couldn't be with me. From first grade on, I was a latchkey kid, often getting to school and back alone. That usually meant taking the bus—or sometimes two or three buses—on winding commutes that had me waiting morning and night in the dark of Seattle winter. My mom taught me to read schedules and timetables, and she'd drill me on the plan—when to leave, where to wait. I learned the importance of all that rehearsing on my very first day of school, when, despite

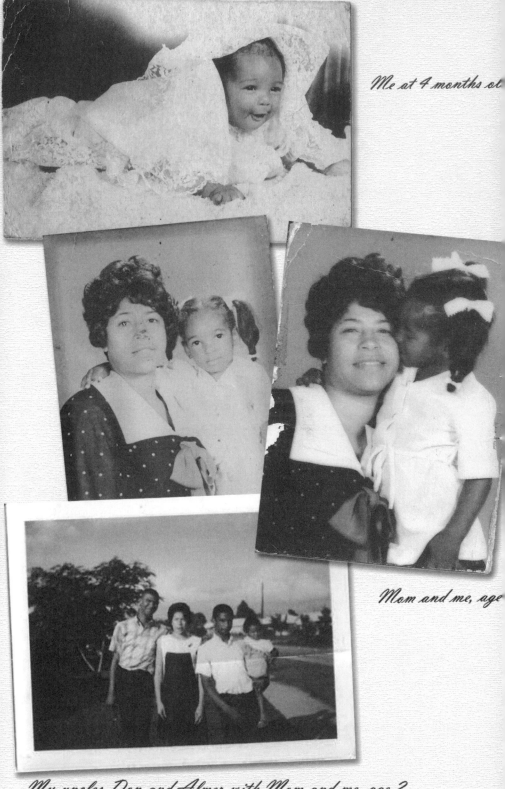

Me at 4 months o[l]

Mom and me, age

My uncles Don and Almer with Mom and me, age 2

having carefully worked out bus numbers and directions, I decided to ask advice of Ammine Berry, the only other black girl in my class and my soon-to-be best friend.

"Listen," she told me with great authority, "just get on the bus that stops in front of the school and it'll get you there. I'll show you." Ammine, I soon learned, rarely let not knowing something prevent her from sounding as if she did. But in that first moment of feeling alone and a little lost, I thought she must be a guide sent from heaven. So two intrepid six-year-olds climbed onto the school bus and got off near Ammine's house—miles in the opposite direction from where I needed to be. That was the last time I let myself climb on a bus without quizzing the driver about our real destination.

I did have occasional babysitters. My uncle Almer, who was a decade younger than my mom, was a navy man stationed in Seattle—he still suspects that Mom had a hand in that—and he'd come stay with us for a week or two when his ship came in. Mom's other brother, Don (he's two years older than Almer), would also visit when his navy travels brought him back to town. Neither asked about our vagabond lifestyle—Mom was the big sister with the place to crash, and as far as they were concerned, it was none of their business if we floated around the city. "All those apartments were nice," Almer says. "I thought La V'onne was just restless."

Almer got a glimpse of my life that not too many others saw. He remembers giving me a ride to school one winter and marveling that when we left at my accustomed time, it felt like the middle of the night, and we arrived before anyone else. "It was so early in the morning, the school was all locked up and dark. It was just you and the janitor," he says. "And you were so small!"

It was that way every day. I'd take a bus that let me off way before the rest of the kids showed up and wait in whatever part of the school was open—sometimes it was with the secretaries outside the principal's office, sometimes the library. I knew all the adults who were working at that hour. And when the janitor opened up my classroom, I'd sit alone and do my homework or read. I was always the first one there.

During the school day I was the driven kid, the one with her hand always in the air, the first one with the answer. I felt as though I'd always known how to read, and math clicked easily in my brain. A French teacher came on Fridays to teach us vocabulary with a bingo game that rewarded the winner with Jolly Rancher candies. The inside of my desk was a candy storehouse—I had a lot of luck and a very good memory.

I liked being the best and fought for it; I was about as alpha as they come. I ran outside playing "capture the flag" with the boys, whispered with the girls, and always had a plan. When we found a dead bird on the playground in first grade, I insisted that our class hold a funeral, complete with a procession to a gravesite on the playground. I, of course, was the priest.

I palled around with a couple of boys—Johnny, my favorite, and pair of girls named Mindy and Wendy. All of them were from families with big homes by the water and maids or nannies who'd make us snacks on the occasions when I could get a ride over to play after school. As the days lengthened in the spring, we'd keep our wide-ranging tag and hide-and-seek games going far into the evening on big lawns that felt like parks, with a froth of blooms on the well-manicured azaleas and camellias opening like giant white moths against glossy green leaves that arched overhead.

But I was closest to Ammine, more for reasons of family status than color. Her life, it turned out, had enough drama to make mine seem almost normal.

"You don't have a father, right?" she observed early on. "That's okay—my parents are separated. I stay with my dad sometimes and my mom sometimes, and I have my stuff at two houses."

"We've had a couple of different houses, too," I said. "It's not bad."

"At least you have your mom all the time," she said, sounding envious. Her mother was white, her father black, and because her mom traveled a lot for business, she was most often at her father's place, where her grandmother would take care of her. Her parents were wealthy, but it didn't seem to change her—she was down-to-earth, more like me. And once we went over to her father's house, I knew things weren't always easy for her. There were hippies hanging out, and he was trying to be one. It was weird, but I didn't make a big deal about it. Neither of us liked explaining our home life to other kids, which made us natural confidantes, and my mom was comfortable letting Ammine come over. For many years she was the only friend I was allowed to bring home.

My "normal" was being home alone. And the routine, whether my mom was there or not, was that there was no routine, no set-in-stone mealtimes or homework time or bedtime or chores. If I was hungry when I got back from school, I knew how to make a sandwich or heat water for Cup-a-Soup or ramen noodles. If I wanted to watch old movies into the night, that was up to me. If I wanted to drop my clothes on the floor when I took them off, no problem. My mom did that, too.

Compared to the other kids, I was being raised by wolves, and luckily, the freedom suited me. But Mom and I did have safety rituals. After she heard me telling someone on the phone that she wasn't available, she began to fret about what might come of my talking to strangers who called while she was out. So we developed some of the few rules in my life: No answering the door when I was home alone. No answering the phone then, either, unless I first heard her signal—two single rings.

In case of an emergency, she insisted that I know her work number, my grandmother's phone number, and our home number. These we worked on after dinner, especially right after a move when there would be yet another new home phone to memorize. For most second or third graders, knowing your phone number and address is rote. For me it was a maddening exercise that wouldn't let me forget how different our life was from that of other families.

I added rituals of my own to make my time alone less scary. TV noise would drown out the sounds of the street and the unnerving creaks of a new place, so I'd flip on the set as soon as I walked in the door and use its laugh tracks, shoot-outs, and talking heads for company. If I were feeling especially nervous, I'd prop a chair under the doorknob till my mom got home. I carried an umbrella for a solid year, rain or shine, after a dog chased me near a bus stop. I wanted to be able to protect myself, and I didn't care what anyone said about my odd habits (to this day I'm uncomfortable around big dogs).

My reward for being more grown-up than kids my age was being treated like a grown-up—I was my mother's closest confidante, the one she laughed and cried with. Romances, finances, moods that swept in like storms from the Pacific—she shared every hope and worry. I was used to being consulted and having a say.

"You liked him, didn't you?" Mom asked. I was sitting on the floor between her legs for my weekly session with the hot comb—oil on my kinky hair, a metal comb heated on the stove and pulled through to straighten it, section by section, in an hour of intimate contact (and peril to the delicate skin of my ears and scalp). We'd gone out to dinner with a new suitor the night before, and Mom was in the glow of "maybe he'll stick around." She dated sporadically, and I was always included in the predate preparations as well as the postdate debriefing.

"He was boring," I said, blunt as ever.

"Don't you say that where he can hear! He's a good man, and he's got that sweet mouth." She gave my hair a tug.

"Mom! I don't want to hear about it." I could imagine the two of them kissing, but I didn't want to.

In our early years of scraping and creative financing, Mom's admirers were a welcome source of distraction as well as affection—and sometimes cash. Almost all of them were a certain type: handsome, nicely dressed, and able to keep up with her forays into politics and work talk. That was no surprise. She'd had one consistent bit of guidance for me from the time I was old enough to arrange weddings for my Barbies: It's as easy to marry a rich man as a poor one. It was a given that Mom would only favor men whose jobs would keep them in shiny Italian shoes, tailored suits, and status cars.

I was both seen and heard when a man came to call, and I went along on enough dates to work out a system with my mom. "Leese, you're going to have to help me tonight," she'd say as she adjusted her skirt in front of the mirror, smoothing it over her curves. "You know how these men are. You let me know if you like this one, and I'll do the same, all right?"

Then with a spritz of Shalimar and a confident swipe of red lipstick, she was ready and we were off.

I loved to watch her in action. On a date, she was effervescent, with the smoothness of a Southern belle and enough cattiness to have an edge that let a man know not to mistake charm for emptyheadedness. It was fine with her if I didn't like someone she was having fun with, but dinner, she made clear, wasn't the place to express it. If I turned sarcastic or confrontational, I'd get a pinch under the table and a walk to the ladies' room, where she'd tell me I needed to turn my attitude around. I've never been good at hiding my feelings.

If it looked as though things were going badly and our date was dull or obnoxious or just simply moving too fast, my mom would give me one of her looks, and I'd develop a terrible stomachache or a "fever" that needed prompt attention. "No, we won't be having dessert—my girl's eyes look so tired, don't they?" A flurry of excuses and apologies would see us to the door, and we'd leave as unencumbered as when we'd walked in. She was highly selective, so my acting was pretty well practiced.

One of Mom's admirers was John Doyle Bishop, the owner of an haute couture boutique on Fifth Avenue that bore his name. Mom had walked into the shop not long after we moved to Seattle, and almost immediately she was modeling in trunk shows and for private customers at the lush modern space—and taking home the bright suits and frothy dresses the flamboyant Irishman occasionally gave her in payment. He adored her and indulged me, letting me sit amid his high-society clients as Mom and the other models circulated through the airy space. She'd dress me up in a frilly dress, white anklets, and shiny patent Mary Janes and put colored ribbons in my hair. I'd watch the shows wide-eyed.

Mom didn't often wear the clothes Bishop gave her, but I liked to riffle through them in her closet, feeling the heft and texture of the fabrics in that one small section of her otherwise functional wardrobe.

We had no money to speak of, but luxury—whether it came in the form of a beautiful dress or dinners at the best restaurants in town—wasn't foreign to us. Mom always found a path to it and, in her way, made sure I had a taste.

Three

Always Moving

One white sofa, long, impractical, and capable of imparting a certain glamor to any sort of apartment

One coffee table

One tabletop color television

Four table lamps

One formal dining room table with four chairs and a buffet

One double bed and nightstand

Two dressers

Two boxes of china, glasses, pots and pans, a handful of spice jars: an instant kitchen

Two boxes of assorted groceries

One small box of cleaning supplies

Two boxes of child's drawings, photos, mementos

Two boxes of toys, dolls, and games

One French Provincial–style four-poster bed with white canopy and gold details on the frame

One wardrobe box of women's clothes

One wardrobe box of girls' clothing

Framed artwork: color studio portrait of a young black girl (me), photo of a black farm couple (my grandparents), photo of a young black mother with daughter (us)

We were a quick, cheap move, an easy load and unload. After a year or so, some of our bulkier pieces of furniture and nonessential belongings like mementos had taken up residence in a storage space, and the rest was simple to pack. We stashed the empty boxes in a closet, and when it was time to tape them together again, I got good at tossing in my things. After a while, neither of us bothered to do much unpacking. Home for me was my four-poster bed from Sears, and once it was set up, I'd pull out a pink baby doll with a music box inside that you could wind up with a tiny key on the back. When it tinkled "Playmate, come out and play with me," I was in my haven, my floating island. If we were in a fancy place, like the huge condo near Lake Union with a balcony and a view of the city, I was thrilled by the change of scene. As often as not, though, our next perch would be far out of town, in Bellevue or Redmond, where rents were cheaper. I learned not to get attached.

"Always moving" was a state of being for us. We couldn't stop, couldn't rest. In my mom's mind, I'm sure much of that had to do with staying ahead of bill collectors and bitter landlords and the chance that someone at work would find out how we were getting by. It was as though we'd been snatched by the winds of a tornado, and somehow we'd be fine as long as we kept spinning. If we stopped to look closely at our precarious state, we'd crash to the ground and have to survey the rubble. So instead we flew on.

Mom looked for new jobs, new houses. I was propelled by the hunt for the next A. According to my mom, I'd need all I could get. "When you're a black female, good isn't good enough," she said, echoing generations of black mothers before her. "You're going to have to work harder and do better, just so people will take you seriously." I took her words to heart. If there was extra credit to be done, I piled it on. I wanted the A-plus, not just the A. The funny thing was that Mom didn't insist. If I'd said I was too tired to do my homework, she'd have told me to rest. She believed in me. I was the one who needed to prove to the world that she was right.

That became a problem when a new student showed up at Epiphany in the third grade. She was a pretty Asian-American girl, shy and brainy. For the first time in my life, I had competition. I'd handily been number one on every test and paper, but suddenly, there was someone who'd best me by a point or two. Some kids might have enjoyed having an equal, a true rival, but I hated it.

Mom couldn't see anything but the As on the papers I brought home, and I think she was surprised by how much the new girl upset me. "Honey," she said when I asked what to do, "nothing beats a winner but a try."

I didn't like the idea that I was not the winner, but I could go with the "try" idea. And try I did. On the playground I lobbied to make sure no one talked to the new girl. "I can't be on your team if you play with her," I pouted to the other kids. I even roped my friends into tactics that had an uncomfortable twinge of *Lord of the Flies.*

"When she walks by, let's whisper, then point at her."

"What do we say?" someone asked.

"It doesn't matter," I said. It didn't. We mumbled gibberish while we giggled in her direction, and she walked away, stricken.

My teacher took me aside and tried to explain that I needed to be friendly to everyone, especially the new girl, but I was only so successful at tempering my resentment. At the end of the year, she transferred to a new school. All these years later, I still feel guilty about that. I've blocked out her name, but I can still see the sadness on her face. Little Asian girl, if you're out there, I owe you an apology.

Even when it agitated me, school was the calm center of our whirlwind, and it remained constant in a way our home couldn't.

Especially in my first years at Epiphany, when all it took to thrive was effort and we kids seemed almost blind to color and circumstance, it was my refuge. Maybe that's why I snapped the way I did when I ran into the bully at the bus base.

We were living in Bellevue then, and I would take one school bus to a transfer point where I'd catch another bus that let me off near my campus. I'd been aware of a loudmouthed kid bothering people, but I'd kept my head down and my nose in a book, and he hadn't singled me out for any attention . . . until the day we were both at the front of the line waiting to get on.

"Hey, chocolate chip!" he snickered.

"What did you say?"

"You heard me, chocolate chip," he said.

I didn't think. I picked up my antidog umbrella and whacked him. And then I whacked him again. "Take it back!" I yelled.

He flung his arms into a roundhouse swing, and we were in a full-on brawl when the bus driver and another adult pulled us apart and marched me over to the office so they could call my mom. I wasn't worried about any bruises or scratches I'd inflicted. But when people began to talk about how I might not be able to take the bus anymore, I panicked. This was serious. I needed to get to school.

My mom had to do some major apologizing to the bully's parents before I was allowed back on the bus that week.

"What got into you?" she asked me.

"He called me a chocolate chip, Mom."

She tried to hide a smile. "And that's why you hit him? What he said wasn't right. It was ignorant, and I understand why you're upset. But you can't hit everybody who calls you a name," she said. "You're not going to do that anymore, do you hear me? A boy like that is not worth it."

He and I didn't tangle again. I'd clutch my umbrella, sit in the front seat of the bus, and let him pass without a word.

I think Mom asked Daddy to talk to me after the bus incident. Daddy was the man in our life, the one who felt like her match—witty, smart as she was. Mom had big, strong hands, not what you'd expect from a woman as feminine as she was, but they looked almost delicate when he held them. She was wild about him. Other men drifted through. Daddy belonged to us. He'd come over in the evenings and help me with my homework or watch TV. Mom seemed to relax around him and even get younger, shrieking into the bedroom as he chased her. He was wealthy—an attorney. Just her type.

But nothing in our life was simple. Daddy was married to someone else. I knew exactly what that meant: No going out with him to our favorite restaurant in Seattle, no talking about Daddy to anyone, ever—even Ammine. The other "no" was "No talking back to Daddy." He was the closest thing I'd had to a father since we'd left my real one behind. Daddy had known me since I was tiny, and if he wanted me to do something—clean the house or go to bed—that was that. We weren't companions and equals like my mom and me. He was Daddy.

We got to go with Daddy to the beach—we met him there and stayed overnight at a hotel—and even went to a party at his house once.

Mom had somehow met Daddy's wife at a social function connected to her job, and the wife had invited us to the party. Mom debated about going, but curiosity got the best of her. She wanted to see that hidden part of Daddy's life, his real one.

She fussed over the way I dressed and repeated her instructions to me on the way over. "This is Daddy's house, this is his party, and you can't be close to him there, understand?" I had to pretend I didn't know him, even though he'd been with us for probably half my life.

I couldn't believe how beautiful his house was. It was as huge as my classmates' homes and so much nicer than any place we'd lived. Fancy furniture. So many rooms. I tried to imagine what it would be like to have the fireplace, the sweep of a living room with a piano at one end, enormous windows with the lake glittering behind them. He had two children of his own who got to be there all the time. I wanted to ask them what he was like with them, but a bigger part of me didn't want to know. I was confused and angry when we left. He had so much money—why couldn't he help us more?

My real father tried to stay in touch. On my birthday a package might appear—one year it was a pretty pink coat. Sometimes there would be a card that Mom would shake open, looking for a check. "We need rent money and he sends a coat," she told me, full of disdain. She'd pushed for child support, but there was nothing coming. Just the packages and an occasional phone call. "It's your father, you want to talk to him?" I'd shake my head vigorously and walk away. Of course I didn't want to talk to him. I'd made my choice when we left. I didn't choose him.

Mom began looking for another job. Even with the moving, non-stop juggling, and checks from Daddy to help out when we skated too close to the edge, there was no way to pretend we could keep going on what the university was paying. The phones stopped working for a while, and when we got them back on, they rang and rang with people wanting money.

It was painfully clear that we weren't ever going to be the ones living in Daddy's big house. Mom talked about breaking up with him, making a fresh start. Instead, she broke up with the university and got into government work, taking a job at the Department of Housing and Urban Development. She broke up with modeling as well that year, when vanity forced her to quit.

Mom subjected me to the singeing and pulling of the hot comb, and I always hoped it would turn out like hers. I loved the silkiness of her long, loose waves and the way they framed her face. She had the beauty I hoped to grow into.

On the "day that changed everything," she'd decided to go to a salon for her first chemical relaxing treatment, a special treat. But as soon as the chemicals were combed through her hair, something went wrong. The hair began to break off all over her head. I screamed when I saw her scalp showing through in patches and the remaining stubs of hair sticking up at odd angles. I know she was traumatized, but almost before she could assess the damage, she had to calm me down. She looked maimed to me, as though she'd lost an appendage.

She wore short, business-like wigs until her hair grew back, and when it did, it was never the same—she never wore it long again. I wouldn't say she lost her confidence then, but that young, sexy Southern belle disappeared, replaced by someone more marked by worry.

I escaped into my own bubble. At the end of third grade, my teacher put us on individual learning programs that let us go at our own pace. Mine was fast, and I could get ahead during my "wait for the bus" hours before and after school or even on the long drive home. My mom indulged me with the toys I clamored for—a model train, a chemistry set. In typical laissez-faire fashion, she let me wind my train through the house, stepping over the tracks that emerged unpredictably from under chairs and tables. The chemistry set came with a microscope and a Bunsen burner, and I was allowed to heat concoctions over the flame. I worked my way through a book of experiments, changing the colors of the liquids in my test tubes again and again like a magician. I'd had an Easy-Bake oven, but something as simple as a light bulb cooking a miniature cake couldn't hold my interest nearly as well as the idea of being a mad scientist, or perhaps an Encyclopedia Brown–style detective, like the kids in the books I devoured. I was the daughter of a professional woman who carried a briefcase and had distanced herself from any expectation that she'd work and do housework and bake cakes. I wouldn't be clamoring for toy kitchens and vacuum cleaners.

For all that, I was a girly girl, too, trooping off to ballet class every Saturday at the Cornish School, climbing the stairs of an old brick building redolent of chalk and what I vaguely labeled "that art smell"—some combination of oil paint and sweat. I loved the discipline of dance and the way my tall, lithe teacher floated across the floor, but for the life of me I couldn't tell right from left in her classes, and counting out steps and beats felt like work the way math problems never would. Like a lot of little girls, I was in it for the costumes—short pink tutus and shiny pink shoes. I know I stood out from the tiny blonde snow princesses, tall for my age and beginning to fill out, but for as long as I clung to the fantasy of dancing, no one dissuaded me.

I didn't feel deprived of anything. Even the dancing ballerina doll I clamored for appeared under the Christmas tree. But when the pivoting leg it spun on broke and we took it in to be mended, I got another reminder of why I should savor every gift that came to me when it appeared. The doll vanished onto the repairman's shelf, and there was never money to get it back. The doll's moment had come and gone: Our lives had whirled on.

Four

Wonder Woman

I had trouble seeing the blackboard when I got to fourth grade, and after I'd asked to change desks a couple of times so I could move closer, my teacher told my mom I needed glasses. The heavy brown frames took over my face. Everything snapped into focus, but it was a decidedly mixed blessing—now I had a twenty-twenty vision of how odd I looked, how different from the perfect little blonde girls sitting all around me. I sized myself up: chubby, dark, four-eyed. I took a cue from Ammine and went for a more sophisticated hair-style, moving my ponytails from the sides to one on top of my head and one below it in back. It was sleeker and it helped, but not a lot.

Ammine and I had spent a couple of weeks at a camp in the San Juan Islands that had A-frame cabins around a lake. I'd learned to sail, and we'd hiked and played epic games of capture-the-flag among enormous trees. That meant I had something to talk about in our first show-and-tells of the year. But something was changing, or perhaps this was the year I was fated to see things I'd been blind to before.

The other kids came back with endless stories of going to Aspen for the music festival or to Europe for the museums, and when they talked about sailing, they didn't mean going out on a little Sun-fish but on a fifty-footer their parents kept in the marina. Even the smartest girl in the class couldn't compete with that, at least not if the game was to match or one-up the experiences of everyone else.

Mom was struggling to find her footing in the government bureaucracy. I suppose I could've regaled my classmates with tales of how cutthroat things were at HUD, and how people were always trying to stab my mom in the back so she couldn't get ahead and how hard she had to work to stay even. Those were the stories she told me when she flopped down dead tired at the end of the day. She was even working Saturdays to keep up with her paperwork, which meant our "fun time" together was limited. We went for long stretches when she was too tired to cook, and we'd started eating a lot of take-out and TV dinners.

As the school year wound on, I began to dread having to come up with something new to share for show and tell. My mom's friend Anne occasionally took me out for an afternoon of Gilbert and Sullivan or ballet, but I began to feel like the only person at the party who hadn't been to Antigua or London with the nanny. Clamming up wasn't an option, and I was too outgoing for that anyhow, so I took a different tack.

I waved my hand for a turn. "I had a really exciting week. We had Kentucky Fried Chicken five times," I said, exaggerating my delivery to the point of sarcasm. "It's finger lickin' good!"

The kids began to titter.

"That's enough, Lisa," my teacher cautioned. But stirring things up was a release for me, and I learned to make jokes, play the clown.

I needed a comic's thick skin—or a rhino's. I had always liked and played with Johnny, and now when we played hide-and-seek, I found myself thinking about him—not as a boyfriend, because no one was really coupling up yet, but as someone I'd consider in that way. I begged my mom for a new outfit to wear on our Friday "free day," the rare opportunity to get out of our uniforms and express ourselves. There had to be Famolare Get Theres, platform sandals with a scalloped "wave" sole, a craze that swept through school from the older kids to the youngest, and I had my eye on white pants and a sunny yellow top. I studied my transformation in the mirror when I put on my lucky outfit. If anything was going to impress Johnny, this would be it.

I strutted into class, and when Mindy and Wendy commented—favorably, I thought—on how unusually bright my clothes were, I let out the secret of my budding crush.

"They told me what you said about, you know, liking me," Johnny said as we were walking in from a game not long after. "We're all friends but don't think I could like you that way. I'm not black like you. What would our kids be like? Maybe they'd be zebras!"

I tried to laugh. And when my mom got home that evening, I cried.

"Oh, honey," she said as she wrapped her arms around me. "It just means he's not the one for you, and he doesn't know what he's missing. When the right person comes along, he'll love you for you, just the way I love you."

I nestled into her and tried to believe that even in matters of the heart, she could make everything all right.

Her own heart was being soothed by a new admirer she'd met at work, a "keeper" I called Uncle Jim, who was as large and jovial as the Cosby character Fat Albert, with a big smile for me and kind eyes that always drifted to Mom. She didn't seem interested in him in that way, but he was good to us—he'd take us to dinner and on outings around town, and unlike Daddy he could be seen with us anywhere; he was proud to have us with him. Uncle Jim cemented his place in my heart the day he saw me choking on a fish bone and reached over without a moment's hesitation to pull it out of my throat. Gifts and nice meals are

great, but to have someone there when you need them—I loved
the way that felt.

Wonder Woman came to my rescue around that time, too. As soon
as I saw Lynda Carter on TV that fall in her superheroine guise,
I worshipped her. I made my own Wonder Woman costume—a
cardboard crown colored with a yellow marker and embellished
with a bold red star; cuffs fashioned from slit toilet-paper tubes
and detailed with Sharpie jewels; a lasso of heavy string; a pillow-
case cape. A girl on the firing line can definitely use magic bullet-
deflecting cuffs, and there's nothing like a Lasso of Truth that can
cut off other people's dissembling—and then make them obey. I
spent hours, both alone and with Ammine, mastering Wonder
Woman's style and stance. I especially liked the way part of her
power came from the way she sprang her identity on the unsus-
pecting. She'd throw her ordinary body into a spin, and when the
top slowed, she was transformed. I spun till I was dizzy, knowing in
some part of my brain that if I didn't turn into Wonder Woman, it
was because I hadn't tried hard enough. My mom had drilled into
me that I could be anything—anything—if I believed in myself as
much as she believed in me.

The only thing easy about that year was schoolwork. My teacher
continued the self-paced learning we'd started in third grade, divid-
ing us into groups so students at similar levels could occasionally
work together on projects. I had my eye on the "platinum" level,
leaving the more pedestrian "red" and "blue" to the other kids. My
mom had bought me math workbooks to help occupy my time

when I was off for the summer, and I was used to solving problems myself. I'd already taught myself some of the basics of fractions, decimals, and long division, and I'd turn in my homework, neat and error free, always asking for more.

Social studies, English, spelling, science experiments, French— I had a platinum-level appetite for the work. You could say it was almost my hobby. When I was "in the zone," just me and the lessons, everything else fell away—the little embarrassments, the terse voices on the phone that always belonged to bill collectors. We went out to the street one afternoon, and the car was gone. I was sure it had been stolen, but Mom got on the phone to Daddy, not the police, to get it back. After that we were never sure—did we just forget where we parked? Or had a repo man come after us again?

Because she didn't believe in hiding anything from me, and we were better as a team, as she always said, I was Thelma to her Louise as we invented ways to keep our heads above water. We made paying the bills a game. Whom would we outsmart? What trick would we use to keep the lights on, the car in the driveway? Before most kids ever had an inkling about how their parents handled their money, I was sealing the envelopes on payments that I knew Mom had scrambled with a bad account number or date or address. I was more cautious than she, and I'd sometimes squeak out an "Are you sure, Mom?" But what choice did we have? I knew my mother well enough to be certain of one thing: If there were a sign right in front of her with big red letters that read, "Don't do it!" she'd most definitely take it as a challenge. She did not believe in defeat, or limits.

I know the strain of all that persevering took a toll on Mom. She retreated into her room with the *Times* after dinner, and I'd find her there, sprawled under the covers, the sheets of newsprint slipping out of her hand and onto the floor as she dozed. On many evenings I'd get up from my homework and go into the bedroom to gather up the paper, help her out of her clothes if she hadn't fully undressed, and turn off the light.

The nights were all mine. I was nocturnal by nature, and with the TV murmuring in the background, I'd lose myself in my schoolbooks, getting up to watch if the Little Rascals or Shirley Temple were on. It wasn't the singing, dancing Shirley I loved but the sweet, plucky Shirley as Heidi, the orphan who could make even her gruff, indifferent grandfather move heaven and earth for her when she was in trouble.

I got so far ahead of my class that I'd lose track of where the "Platinums" were, so I was glad when we worked together. One project, for social studies, I think, involved building a dwelling of some sort, and I decided mine would be a dollhouse. Mom promised that she'd help me find cardboard and craft supplies, but a couple of days before my house was due, she was frazzled, and I realized I would have to use what was on hand. Painstakingly, I cut walls, windows, doors, and floors from sheets of yellow legal paper and figured out how to tape everything together and make it stand. Even with extra tape at all the seams, the house—all three stories of it—was rickety, but if I held my hand against an outside wall of folded paper, it seemed to be all right.

In class, though, my paper dollhouse sagged next to the fancy, store-bought-looking constructions the other kids brought in. It wasn't hard to guess who'd had help, whose dad was an architect. My teacher was extra encouraging to me, but I could tell she was taken aback by my lined, canary-yellow walls, which were listing like a wet paper bag by the time I got down the hall to class. The other girls had real dollhouses, and they looked nothing like this. My mom always said my best would be more than good enough, but this time I knew it wasn't, even though I got an A.

I retreated into my workbooks.

By Christmas, with no fanfare or even any real acknowledgment, my teacher was slipping me fifth-grade work, and sometime in the spring she and I began to realize that by the time everyone else was wrapping up their fourth-grade lessons, I'd have polished off fifth grade, as well. Inadvertently, I'd found a way to take away a huge burden—I'd saved us a whole year of tuition.

"What are you saying?" my mom asked when my teacher called her in.

"I don't think there's any question—she needs to skip a grade," my teacher said. "I don't have anything else to give her."

For the first time that year, I felt like my old self, the certified leader of the pack. But when I let Ammine in on what was happening, she was livid.

"You mean we're not going to be together for fifth?" she said. "I thought we were friends! Why do you always have to show off like that?"

The school administrators seemed to be in Ammine's camp. I might be intellectually ready for sixth grade, they told my mom, but there were other considerations. Sixth was a transitional year, and socially, I might suffer.

Mom went ballistic. "Do they expect me to believe that if you were a little white girl from one of those wealthy white families we would even be having this discussion?" she vented to Daddy. "What do they want her to do, spend a whole year pretending she's not as smart as she is? You know what this is about," she said. "You and I know very well what this is. They don't want a little black girl skipping past their white children. How are they going to explain to the other parents that my child is superior? They just can't stand it. And they are not going to get away with it."

But the school elders wouldn't budge, and my teacher was beside herself. Mom decided to take me elsewhere. The good news was that Lakeside, one of the most elite prep schools in town, was willing to let me start the next school year in sixth grade, with the caveat that they'd spend a few months evaluating my "readiness." The bad news was that Lakeside was a lot more expensive than Epiphany. Even with a scholarship, it would be a stretch to make it work.

The only person who seemed to feel any kind of pure joy for me was Uncle Jim. When he heard the news, he beamed the way the grandfather in *Heidi* did when he was reunited with Shirley. I put on my fancy white pants, yellow top, and Get Theres and we piled into the car for lunch at the Space Needle. Sitting in the revolving restaurant, I was on top of the world. I felt just like Wonder Woman.

FIVE

Moods and Secrets

Mom was always singing R&B tunes or practicing a hymn. Around the house, and especially in the car, we'd join in with the radio, caught up in our own duets.

Whitney Houston would soar along, reliving her "stolen moments," and Mom and I would sail in tandem to the last "Saving all my love for you."

Mom had been in a choir in Haynesville, and at the black church we attended in Seattle, she was a star. She had a beautiful voice. Our minister, a handsome family man, doted over her when he saw her at services and choir practice, putting a friendly arm around her shoulder and drawing "Sister La V'onne" into conversations, making sure she had a solo.

He started coming over to our house to check in on us, and almost immediately I knew those visits had nothing to do with prayer or counseling or some gift of fellowship. I could tell that he was interested in Mom the way Daddy was and that she was sizing him up, trying to keep a respectable distance while she figured out if there was something he could do to help us. I'd say hello to him at the door and then move to another part of the house, leaving them to do whatever it was that they needed to. I was familiar with the man-woman game by that time, and I knew when to stay out of the way. I didn't want to alienate him because maybe Mom wanted to keep him around.

They may have gone out a couple of times, but Mom quickly reined things in. "I don't want you to disappear," she told me before one of his visits. "I want you to stay right here with me, okay?" The conversation that day stayed focused on choir and my classes, but Mom was warm and attentive to the pastor, too.

It didn't take long for the whispering to start. Maybe our minister's attentions publicly crossed the line, and the church ladies couldn't allow the flirtation to continue. His wife may well have complained. At Sunday school one week, I got into a skirmish with a kid who called Mom a name—it might've been "harlot"—and from then on, I had to sit alone in a pew during the adult service while Mom was with the choir. Before long, the "tsks" and stares got to be too much, and we left the church entirely.

The singing stopped for a while. A young, single mom catches a man's eye, and it's her fault when he pursues the attraction. There was something wrong with that. A minister was supposed to help protect vulnerable people like us, not make us more so. Mom was stung, and Daddy was no comfort at times like this. He didn't want to hear about other men.

But Whitney Houston knew the story of how hard it is to live on your own. We let her sing our blues.

At the worst of times, when men seemed to be just one more complication in her too-complicated life, Mom would despair. She worried endlessly about finances, but it was man trouble that sent her spinning down. She tried to break things off with Daddy many times, and after a while I'd recognize the signs that it had happened again. A bottle of whiskey pulled from a paper bag on the table, streaked makeup, drapes pulled shut in the bedroom before dark, and her with a drink at her side, crying. She never drank except at times like this, and my heart would seize when I saw her pick up the glass.

I'd try to snuggle up next to her, but I couldn't really get close. She was far away, and even as she tried to explain things to me, I knew she was talking to herself.

"Everything I've tried has gone wrong," she'd say. "I wanted to make a good life for us, but it's just too hard. It would be better if I were just gone." Sometimes she'd add: "I wish I was dead." At the sound of those words she'd cry harder, and I'd feel my chest tighten. What would I do without her?

"I could do it," she'd repeat as if she were working out a plan. "That would solve everything. You could go to your grandmother."

I'd had a recurring nightmare ever since I could remember. A plane would fall from the sky, and I'd be frozen on the ground, knowing my mother was on board, engulfed in flames. The plane crashed night after night, and each time I was helpless. I'd wake with my pulse racing. I couldn't save her.

But talk of death was not a plane crash, and this was not a dream in which I'd scream a scream that caught in my throat and wouldn't leave my mouth. I could rescue her; at least I thought I could. I clutched her hand and pleaded. "Please, Mom, please. You have me, and we have each other. We're going to be okay. We can't give up now—we're going to make it. You'll see. We're going to make it." I said it in as many ways as I could. "Don't leave me, Mom. Let me sleep next to you to be sure you don't leave." Then I tried to make her laugh, or at least smile. I couldn't imagine my life without her, and I had to keep her with me.

If I talked long enough, she'd quiet down and slide into a deep sleep as I sat watching over her, and when she woke, she'd clear away the bottle and the glass. The mood had passed. We'd go on.

Some people would say that it's the parents' duty to shelter their children from the harshness of life, the swoops and swoons of love and hope and money, but I knew Mom's openness, even when it bared her pain, was what brought us closer. I knew her as she really was, flawed and frail and generous. If that knowledge was a burden, I was happy I could carry it. She didn't have to be strong for me—we could be strong for each other.

When things got particularly bad at work, or during one of those long, hard seasons when money wouldn't stretch and every day seemed to hold another slap, a different sort of darkness would descend on my mother. When we moved from a large townhouse in Seattle to a small, noisy building in Bellevue, we both knew there was more to come and that our next move would be sooner than the last. We didn't even bother to unpack anything but our clothes and enough kitchen gear to let us do some easy cooking. When a truck pulled up one weekend afternoon and two men came in to take away the sofa, it was as though we'd expected it so long we hardly blinked. We lounged on the beds and lived around the dining room table.

I thought we'd settled into our new normal—more tentative than before but still anchored by my studying and her job at HUD. Mom came home from work one day, though, and uncharacteristically began railing about the "goddamn mess.""We're living like pigs in here," she yelled. "I can't find a damn thing—just look at this." "This" was a pile of papers spilling across the table onto some dishes from breakfast, the same pile that we always let accumulate without much concern. On a typical day housework was the last item on the to-do list, the one that most often got pushed to tomorrow or next week or never. We were blind to the chaos. But not now.

Mom flung open closet doors and pulled drawers so hard they barely stayed on their runners, slamming them shut with disgust. "We are going to clean up this place once and for all, do you hear me?" she yelled. "You start with your room, and then I want you to scrub that bathroom till it shines."

She crashed her way through the apartment, banging pots into pans as she put things away in the kitchen and scooping up piles of clothes from her bedroom floor, then sending a fistful of hangers flying as she pulled them off the rod. I could've joked about the White Tornado sweeping through, but the crash and clatter of her temper were terrifying enough aimed at the house. I didn't want that fury coming at me. I worked as fast as I could and tried to stay out of her way. If no one was coming over and she insisted on a major cleanup, I knew things weren't going to go well.

I held my breath as she inspected my work. She was still dressed in her work clothes, which were wrinkled now and streaked with dust. She caught a glimpse of herself in the mirror and swore. But the place looked as neat as when we moved in, and I thought the storm would subside. Maybe this time we could look around and admire our work. Maybe she'd calm down.

But Mom wasn't done. She needed to get out of the house— now!—and I would go with her. She changed her clothes and fixed her disheveled office coif.

"Come on, Lisa Marie. I can't wait all day. Look at you half dressed—you only have one shoe on. Get the other one, and let's go."

I hunted for my shoe. In the cleaning frenzy I'd tossed it somewhere, and now I couldn't remember where.

She stood impatiently at the door of my room. I crawled to the edge of the bed and peered under, then dug around the floor of the closet, trying to uncover the shoe without making a mess again. I should've known where it was. It was all my fault.

"Why can you not do the simplest things?" she said. Her voice was rising. I sat amid the toys and sneakers, where it was still quiet, still peaceful.

"That's enough, Lisa," she said in a tone that told me what was coming next. "Go get the belt."

A long, slim belt of black leather always hung on a hook in her closet. It wasn't something I remember her wearing; it seemed to exist solely for the purpose it would be put to now. Two or three times a year, her patience would snap—she would snap—and a hyper bout of cleaning would set the stage for its appearance.

I'd hidden the belt once, but not well enough, and she was enraged when she found it. I'm not sure why I didn't just destroy it, but I think I knew even then that her punishment didn't depend on this totem. My grandmother had used a switch on her. Mom wasn't stupid. If there were no belt, she'd have used whatever was handy, something with more sting than her hand.

"You know what to do, so get to it," she said, the belt now draped over her palm. "Take off your clothes."

We were both in her room now, and I pulled off my skirt and top and underclothes, then reached down to remove my socks. I tried to pile everything carefully, and I tried not to cry.

I folded my arms over my chest to cover myself and turned my back to her. My legs shook as she stepped up behind me.

The belt came down hard on my back. It hit me there again, then landed on my buttocks. My skin burned. I bit my lips, clenched my eyes shut, and tried to hold everything in.

When she started yelling, it was like a volcano erupting. "I do everything for you, and it's only me here to take care of it all. I can only do so much, and you always need more and more. It's only you that I'm doing this for, do you understand me?"

She whaled away on my back and buttocks as I folded in on myself, trying to make myself smaller, but it only made me a better target. When I couldn't stand, she told me to lie across the bed, and she brought the belt down again. "I do everything I can for you, and you repay me with this," she hissed. "I try so hard. Maybe I should send you to your dad and he can do a better job with you."

Her words struck more fear in me than the blows. I understood that we were in a difficult situation and she was doing more than humanly possible to get us through it. She never took vacations, she labored to keep up with everything for her job—politics, the news—she worked long, long hours. This life we had was all-important to her and to me. "You can just go live with your grandma or your father if this is too hard for you," she told me whenever times got tough. It wasn't a threat, it was an open door to something easier. She didn't give me an out to complain. I knew I was with her by choice.

The belt came down and down, and when I finally began to cry, it was less because of the pain than my fear that she'd give up on me and send me away. I'd been to Haynesville, and it wasn't what I wanted. The kids I'd met had accents that made them sound backward—they were nothing like me or the quick, articulate kids at my school. I didn't know my father. I didn't think he was a bad man; he was just someone who wasn't right for my mother, and I knew he wasn't right for me, either. The life he had wasn't what I wanted.

My mom was sure of it, and I was, too. I wouldn't let anyone sentence me to that.

"Please, Mommy," I sobbed. I curled up in a ball and she finally let the belt slide from her hand. Then she started sobbing, too. Her lashing had broken the skin, and welts were beginning to rise, crisscrossing my ribs and the flesh of my buttocks. She touched the marks softly. No one would ever see them—my arms, struggling to shield my naked front, were always held out of the way, and she never struck my legs. I'd stay covered up around other kids until I healed. It was another of our secrets.

Mom wept as she dabbed my wounds with alcohol, and it was as though someone else's hand had done the damage. "Honey, I'm so sorry," she'd say. "Let me make this better." As she nursed me, she'd try to cheer me up. "What do you want to do, see a movie? Go out for something to eat?" Even weak and shaky as I was, I brightened at the knowledge that I'd be in for special treatment—the good kind—for the next few days.

And then she'd start crying again. "You should go to your dad," she'd decide. "I'm not fit to take care of you."

I turned and tried to comfort her. "No, it's okay, Mom. We can do it. We have to stick together."

No matter what, no matter how bad things got, we were a team.

Six

Angel with a Briefcase

Lakeside at first glance was a sea of tall, thin girls with long, blonde hair and boys with cute, perfect smiles. People had been right about the leap from fourth grade to middle school. These tribes of flirting teens and almost-teens weren't just older, they were more outspoken and free-spirited than the little kids at Epiphany, with no uniforms but the jeans and T-shirts they slouched into with perfect cool. At another, larger school I might've just tried to hide out for a while to get my bearings, but Lakeside, with one big brick building and no sprawling wings, was even more contained than my old school. Besides, there's no real place to hide when you're the new kid in classes with just eight or ten students—and the only black girl in the place.

Most of the kids knew each other from at least the year before—the middle school ran from fifth grade to eighth—and some had been on the same prep school path since kindergarten. Their parents seemed to be either hippies or very conservative (which explained the preppie strain that ran through some of the cliques), but all of them were rich enough to afford the kind of tuition and fees that buy things like computer resources for a young Bill Gates, a soon-to-be-famous Lakeside alum who was just starting Microsoft the year I arrived.

Everyone knew my story: I was the one who had three months to prove herself or be sent back to fifth grade. The girl with the briefcase. I'd seen my mom carrying one all my life, and when she asked me if I wanted a backpack for school, I pleaded instead for an attaché, that working woman's badge of seriousness. I did homework on the bus, so I could use it for a writing surface. And I'd have more papers to carry now that I was in middle school. Never mind that no one else would be seen with anything they couldn't sling over a shoulder—the briefcase was me. It meant business.

I was an odd little duck who longed to fit in, but I kept thinking I could do it on my own terms. And sometimes I was just too over-the-top. Before school started, my grandmother sent me an outfit that I adored—an Elle Woods–worthy Pepto-Bismol-pink dress with a matching jacket trimmed in fluffy pink fur. It closed with long ties that dangled huge, pink Marabou pom-poms. When I tried it on and told my mom I planned to wear it to class, she put her foot down and wisely insisted that it wasn't appropriate. I nodded, then stuffed the ensemble into a bag and changed at school. I looked fabulous in the restroom mirror—part Jackie Kennedy, part corporate lawyer, I thought—but as soon as I got into the hall, I realized my mistake. Kids pointed and laughed, and in less than five minutes I was back in a girls' room stall pulling it off and trying to pretend my faux pas had never happened.

Looking back, I'm surprised (and very grateful) that anyone accepted me. It no doubt helped that academically I was at the head of the pack. I was so accustomed to setting a quick pace for myself that I kept right on studying as I had in the final year at Epiphany, putting in extra hours after school while I waited in the library for my mom or the bus and cruising into late-night sessions with the books once my mother had gone to sleep. As at Epiphany, I arrived early, stayed late, and got to know the staff and teachers who opened and closed up the school. But this time I also had the company of a handful of kids who waited with me. They became my closest friends.

Paige, a lean, athletic girl with long brown hair, staked out a spot in the library every day after school. So did Corinne, who'd lived in France for a year and seemed more advanced than Paige and I in the girl-boy department—she quickly had a boyfriend, and she brought back colorful dispatches from the romance front. For all her worldliness, though, she was happy to join Paige and me in our favorite activity: playing "Charlie's Angels" in the empty corridors and grounds of the school after the library closed. There was no set plot for our capers, just variations on "He's hiding over there—let's stake it out!" and "Let's get him!" I got to know every inch of the school because I was the smart Angel, Sabrina, who figured out the logistics that sent us running. Corinne, of course, was Jill, Farrah Fawcett's sexy Angel, and Paige was Kelly, "the sensitive one."

It was liberating to play games in which the only currency was imagination. I had a surplus of that. Paige had everything else, including vacations and a fairy-tale bedroom with a huge bay window. Books, toys, piles of stuffed animals—her sanctum lacked for nothing, and a household staff kept everything in perfect order. But fantasy was our equalizer. As Angels who preferred our own scenarios to most of the teen dramas that surrounded us, we were sisters.

We did have one boy in our midst: Ned, a tall, shy boy who joined us on the steps of the neighboring cathedral when the janitors locked up the main building of the school. We'd hang out there until we had to leave. Sometimes we'd try the church doors and sneak in for a few breaths of the cool, still air, our eyes adjusting to the stained-glass light. Ned knew not to talk if we got inside. I think he could tell it wasn't a joke for me. I craved the feeling I got there, the calm sense of encountering some kind of larger presence and not being alone. I think there must've been something in my expression that gave that away.

I could tell that he sort of liked me, but I'd tasted infatuation at the end of fourth grade, and I knew that Ned wasn't the one for me. I'd gotten close to my bus driver's son on the long rides back and forth to Epiphany when we were the last stops on the route, two murmuring voices in the dark. The little tingle I felt when we touched hands made me want to talk to him on the phone the summer before Lakeside. Ned, though, was just Ned. No tingle, just a cheerful, nerdy lump of boy. I thought of myself as a cool nerd. With Ned I wasn't so sure about the cool.

Every day I missed Ammine, even though we weren't officially speaking because she was so miffed at me for forsaking her at Epiphany. She, at least, would have understood what it was like to get a nonstop stream of clueless questions from otherwise smart people. To Paige and Corinne I was just me—I didn't ask them about being white, and they didn't make anything of my being black. We didn't really seem to see color. But The Questions flowed in from other kids.

"Why is your hair like that?" was a big one. "How come you don't talk like the people on *Good Times*?" was another. *Good Times* was the popular Norman Lear comedy about a black family trying to get by in a Chicago housing project, and the grinning son played by Jimmie Walker punctuated his boasting with "Dyno-MITE!" I cringed when a fake jive-talking Dyno-MITE was lobbed my way at school. I'd taken my cues from a more refined TV model: Diahann Carroll on *Julia*, who played a polished nurse rearing a son alone—and looked like a model as she navigated a world like mine. But with *Good Times* and *Sanford and Son* and *All in the Family* in the air, stereotypes were out in full force, even when the shows that offered them up were mocking them. Dyno-MITE! Right.

Equally annoying was the question about why the only other black student at our school wasn't my boyfriend. "Why?" I wanted to say. "Because he doesn't like me and I don't like him."

Then there were the parents who'd let me have sleepovers with their kids but say things like: "We were thinking about having steak for dinner, but maybe you'd rather have Kentucky Fried Chicken or watermelon or something?" I restrained myself from snapping back with "And maybe you think my mother is Aunt Jemima?" But at home I was always asking my mom: "Why do they have to say things like that? Why are there people who think that because of your color you're less of a human being?"

"Honey, it's lack of education, just not knowing people," she'd say. She helped me understand that the questions were innocent, and it was our job to show people what black women could be— intelligent, articulate, beautiful, witty. Not slangy or uneducated or pregnant teen "welfare queens." One of my cousins had had a baby before she was fifteen, and that was a sore subject.

"'Let's get down!' is not who you are, Leese," Mom said when she saw me trying to clown around to be popular. "That's not what black is—that's just uneducated. You're better than that."

She drilled into me that I would always be judged by the way I looked, the way I spoke. That's why I was at Lakeside. And that's why I'd grown up wearing my hair in two neat, straight ponytails tied up in satin ribbons instead of multiple ponytails or braids or puffs or an Afro. Wanting to be polished, even in middle school, didn't mean I didn't want to be black, just that I was always conscious about the impressions I was leaving, especially on people who didn't have much contact with people like me. I wanted to be in the game, and I knew who was writing the rules. It was polish that got the points.

By December I was officially a member of the sixth-grade class, and for the first time I could relax into being at Lakeside. Being friends with Paige helped. She and I were together in every class except foreign language—I was still taking French, but she was in Latin—and we shared a crush on our math teacher, a handsome young man who could make algebra exciting. We made a point of lingering with some of his other "fans" to ask questions after class, even when I didn't have any.

My reputation as a smart kid got a boost when I came in second in a big spelling bee (and yes, I remember the word that was my downfall: develop. In the clutch I froze, then sputtered out a final "e," making it a little more French but a lot less correct). I still had the hand-in-the-air urgency I'd always taken to class with me, and once kids got to know me, I was voted "most likely to succeed" at yearbook time.

"That's the kiss of death, you know," my mom told me with a laugh, but I know she was proud. I was just glad to have an identity there. If I couldn't win "prettiest" or "best smile," I was okay with success.

Mom and I did all right for most of my first couple of years at Lakeside. With my scholarships and Mom's promotions, we only had to move a couple of times. I remember eating a lot of Chinese food, one of those small, telling signs that we were solvent enough for regular restaurants and didn't have to pick up fast food or wait for Daddy or Uncle Jim to take us out. Our apartments stayed constant—two bedrooms, nice neighborhoods, mostly in Bellevue, and a phone that was quiet not because it had been disconnected but because the creditors were hounding someone else.

Mom still couldn't bring herself to scrimp on the extras that come with private school life, so I spent a few weeks at a nice little camp with Paige and some other girls from school, and I kept up with ballet, graduating to a longer tutu and toe shoes stuffed with lamb's wool. Adolescence hadn't done anything for my grace. My breasts developed early and between feeling unbalanced by their heft and trying to hunch to minimize them, I was, if anything, even more clunky. I'd never lost my right-left confusion, so now I was dancing with a band on my leg to distinguish one side from the other.

Still, Mom pulled money out of her wallet for costumes and Cornish School tuition, and she applauded at my recitals no matter how I did. We both knew ballet would never be my forte, but we were both in love with the idea of it, the romance. She had an image in her mind of a classic education—and it came with tutus, ivy-covered brick buildings, and summers of camping, sailing, and roasting marshmallows with scions of the wealthy. She might not have put it quite that way, but that's the package she always tried to wrap up for me.

In seventh grade I wasn't just the briefcase girl but the one earning A-pluses for things like a detailed timeline showing the battles of the *Iliad* and the *Odyssey* and the world events surrounding them. We were way ahead of our public school peers. But perhaps the most lasting lesson that year came from one infamous party—a private, "everyone's invited" event at the massive home of a girl named Tina. The word was that there would be slow dancing, something that was still new to me, and I asked my mother to show me how to do it.

"Slow dancing?" she said. "There's not much to it. Most of the time all you need to do is sway."

Mom drove me to Tina's, warning me not to let some boy get too close and repeating the mantra she'd started using when I got my first bra: "Don't let him touch you there!" I leaned my head against the window, trying to push my ear into a crack where the air whistled past so I could drown out the lecture. She was wide open about sex, and she'd never been modest, walking around the house nude or half-dressed. But somehow that made the whole business of sex seem like something that belonged to her. Which was fine with me—I didn't want to do it, and I really didn't want to hear about it. I'd even tried not to let her know when I'd gotten my period the year before—it was all vaguely embarrassing.

Paige saw us pull up and met me at the door. Kids were spilling out onto the lawn, and it looked as though the whole class had shown up. "Her parents are gone, and her brother's got pot," Paige told me in a rapid whisper when my mom had driven off. "And there's kissing."

"Let's not do it," I said. "We'll get in trouble." We walked through the house. The lights were low in every room but the kitchen and the main living room, where the stereo was blasting "Dancing Queen" and Marvin Gaye. It looked like a "regular" party, partly for the benefit of parents who were dropping kids off. "That's the bedroom," someone said, pointing upstairs. Couples were holding hands or had their arms around each other as they slid through the door to the dark room and quickly pushed it shut. "I don't think we should do it," we repeated to our friends, but some were already entwined and disheveled. Sneaking off to kiss was one of the main events. Slow dancing, as promised, was another.

We walked into the dim room where the ballads were playing and stood against the wall, watching. Mom was right—there was a lot of swaying. Feet hardly moved, but the older boys' hands were covering a lot of ground. Ned appeared next to me, and I thought he might make some kind of funny remark, but instead, he asked me to dance. I glanced over at Paige who mouthed, "Oh, go on!"

"Sure," I told Ned. I clasped my fingers behind his neck as some of the other girls were doing with their partners, keeping my arms more straight than bent to put some distance between us. He rested his big hands gently on my hips. We moved slowly, as though the air were water, and what I remember most is that Ned was sweaty and nervous and breathing on me as he gradually pulled me closer. He was a worse dancer than I was a ballerina. We lumbered.

"Thanks, that was nice," I said, backing away as soon as the song ended. That was as much slow dancing as I could take.

Paige and I ate and drank Cokes and wandered toward the pungent smell of the pot Tina's brother and his friends were smoking. They passed crudely rolled joints—I learned the word that night, along with "roaches"—and they inhaled deeply. We tried to be nonchalant as we stared. We didn't even know any kids who smoked cigarettes.

The class couldn't stop buzzing about the party on Monday. Nor could the parents who heard about their seventh graders being exposed to sex and marijuana. The resulting furor ended unsanctioned class parties and led to a series of "scared straight" assemblies and lectures about the dangers of drugs. For me there was one more bit of fallout—love notes from Ned, who started slipping them into my locker. I was sad they weren't from someone I actually had a crush on, but I was flattered nonetheless, and I saved the letters in a box.

"What should I do, Mom?" I asked as we drove across the floating bridge to my bus stop.

"Just be nice to him, Leese," she said. "You two can be friends, can't you?"

I began to read the letters to her on our trips in, and sometimes we couldn't keep from laughing. "Did he leave you anything today," she'd ask, and I'd pull out the latest. At last I had girl talk to share with her.

Ned was crushed when I finally told him that no, I couldn't be his girlfriend, just his friend. I guess I was his first love. Mine wouldn't come along for five more years. I clung to the world where I was the smart Angel and the only thing to worry about was outsmarting imaginary bad guys.

SEVEN

Betrayal

"We will find a way." That was my mother's mantra, and I always wound up believing it, no matter how far we'd fallen. Near the end of seventh grade, we moved from a comfortable duplex in Bellevue to a small apartment that felt more like a claustrophobic motel suite than our usual homes. When Mom said she had to go off for training for her new job at the Equal Employment Opportunity Commission and that it would last several weeks, I suspected that there was something she wasn't telling me. I wondered (though I never asked or found out) if something had caught up with her and she was being sent off to some sort of rehab, or even jail.

She left me in the care of an older couple from our church whom I recognized but didn't really know, and I stayed in their house near my school. I couldn't detect any difference in Mom when she got home, and I chastised myself for losing faith in her. The truth was, I was happy to go back to our free-form life. My caretakers had been neat and clock-obsessed, with set mealtimes, a punishingly early bedtime, and not a trace of flexibility when it came to household chores. The chaos I had with Mom may have been stressful at times, but it was comfortable, too—it suited us.

Our stars realigned when the school year ended and we abruptly left the "motel" to move to Redmond, a town eight miles northeast of Bellevue. This time the surprise was breathtakingly good. Mom settled us into a huge L-shaped home on a cul-de-sac full of families and children—our first suburb and our first real house. It'd be a long, long ride from my school in the fall, but I couldn't complain. We now had a huge living room with white carpeting and a fireplace, and we could sprawl into what felt like acres of space, inside and out. We had a dining room, a huge kitchen, even an extra bedroom. I rode my bike past the tall pines and maples that lined our street, and I marveled that a milkman delivered not just milk but my favorite mint chocolate chip ice cream. To our door.

For once I could walk out on an afternoon and find someone to play with—and for the first time ever, Mom was happy to let me bring home kids I knew from school. This was a place with potential. I put flyers in every mailbox on the cul-de-sac advertising my babysitting services, and Mom helped me follow up, walking door to door with me to meet the parents and vouch for me. I made a small fortune taking care of the street's gaggle of babies, along with a couple of eight- or nine-year-olds, whom I'd watch when their parents needed relief. The kids my age would come to keep me company, and my jobs turned into ready-made opportunities for socializing.

Emmett ruined everything. He just appeared one day, a tall, handsome guy with chiseled features, light brown skin, and big brown eyes. Mom stood close to him, leaning into his arm. He was young, years younger than she was—and not at all as distinguished as Daddy or even Uncle Jim. He was such an odd fit for her that I left them to each other and didn't make much of an effort to find out his story. Why invest time in a guy who'd be gone before I'd figured out how many Ms and Ts he had in his name?

But Emmett surprised me. He kept coming back.

A navy cook, he'd show up in his short-sleeved khaki shirt and dark pants, rumpled, not spit-shined like my uncles. He'd always gravitate to the kitchen, which must've felt like a friendly outpost in hostile territory once I started making comments to let him know what a lightweight I thought he was. I could see that Mom liked him, and I got that he was attractive, but I didn't understand the symbiosis. Daddy still came around, and the spark between him and Mom made sense to me. But Emmett? To my twelve-year-old eye, he was a big dork. He didn't seem up to my mom's level of intelligence, and he liked to talk about TV or the guys on his ship, not politics or her work. His humor was off, and he seemed out of place with us.

I couldn't figure out his angle. I was sure that he was somehow on the take, and I felt like Tatum O'Neal in *Paper Moon*, when her father picks up Trixie, the circus performer/stripper. Tatum knows that Trixie is going to con her con-man dad, and she knows that he can't see it because Trixie's blinded him with romance. That's what was happening in my very own house, and it galled me all the more that Emmett had shown up just in time to spoil the best setup Mom and I had ever had.

I got plenty of pinches under the table for mouthing off to him, but Emmett himself seemed to take it in stride. He wasn't all bad. When he cooked spaghetti for me, I couldn't help noticing how good and tangy it was. I even might have smiled. Soon he was making it all the time or taking us out for pizza. I knew he was trying to buy me, but I wasn't being bought—the spaghetti strategy was too unsophisticated to improve our relationship, especially after he made a comment about how healthy it was for a girl like me to have meat on her bones. I was no fool. I knew that meant I was fat—and that put him squarely on my enemies list. But at least while I was chewing, I couldn't talk back to him, and I'm sure he took that as a plus.

As much as I expected that if Mom remarried I'd have a doctor or lawyer father, I wasn't bothered at all that Emmett was a cook. But I couldn't stand the way he carried himself. Even Mom would prod him to straighten up from his slouch and tell him to "stop laughing like a donkey." A boyfriend who brayed—he couldn't possibly last. But somehow, he did.

My classes that year are a blur. I know I cruised through everything but U.S. history (a B!) and that there was something about the word problems in math that tripped me up. But most everything was overshadowed by the big announcement early in the fall: Mom and Emmett were getting married.

Mom knew me well enough not to announce the engagement while Emmett was there.

"I want you to be happy for me," she told me. "I know you two are like oil and water, but Emmett will be good for us, you'll see."

I tried not to cry. "He's too goofy for you, Mom," I said.

The light went out of her eyes, and I thought she'd send me for the belt. But all she said was, "This is not your decision to make, Lisa. He's a good man. We're going to make the best of this, and you'll see—it'll be good for all of us." She had the same tight smile on her face that I'd seen when we'd gone on dates because I knew we needed money, and she wasn't seeing Daddy. I'd always been struck by the way she could warm it up when a man she needed was looking and how much it seemed like a grimace when he looked away.

If Mom and Emmett had a wedding, I've blocked it out. Maybe they asked me to be a part of it and I said no. Maybe they just signed papers at the courthouse because I objected so much. I wouldn't be surprised if I'd insisted that I'd raise my hand and say I had "just cause why they may not be lawfully joined together." Given the opportunity, there was no way I'd hold my peace about it. But in my memory, there's no ceremony, no dress, not even a toast to the couple at dinner. The only evidence of the marriage was Mom's new ring.

Denial was my go-to coping strategy. Even when Emmett's clothes took up residence in Mom's closet, I refused to believe that this crazy idea of hers would turn into something permanent. Living happily ever after as a family couldn't be the point of this whole thing—the marriage was a bargain between them, reached without my approval, and it was doomed. All I had to do was wait.

Emmett and his goofy grin shipped out, and I thought that was that. Mom and I were back to normal. She was moving up at EEOC, I was polishing my "most likely to succeed" reputation at school, and I had a band of neighborhood kids to ride bikes with. Every day I looked around our fancy new house and counted my blessings. In a few weeks I began to wonder what all the Emmett fuss had been about. He was just another blip on the screen.

We settled into our usual routine as though nothing had happened. On the long drive into Seattle in the mornings, Mom and I still sang. We'd always been fans of shows with single parents and kids—*Julia* when I was really little, then *The Courtship of Eddie's Father,* and now *One Day at a Time,* with Bonnie Franklin trying to stay ahead of Mackenzie Phillips and Valerie Bertinelli. "Our song" was the theme from *Eddie's Father,* a bouncy Harry Nilsson tune called "Best Friend" that seemed to describe the tight-as-super-glue bond between us. Now that I was practically a teenager, we felt much more like best friends to me than simply mother and daughter. I knew from talking to Paige that that made Mom stand out from other parents even more than her jerry-rigged financial schemes. "She tells me everything," I bragged to Paige.

But when Emmett returned in the spring, I realized I'd been duped. Over one of Emmett's spaghetti dinners, I could see Mom teaming up with him. "We have something we want to tell you," Emmett said.

"We." I hated that word coming from him. They were holding hands, and their interlocked fingers rested on the table. I had to look away.

"Leese, honey," said Mom, "I'm going to have a baby."

My gaze snapped back, and I stared at them, mind racing. This was some kind of mistake. Why Emmett? Mom didn't need him now—she was doing great at work. She was too old to have a baby. What was she doing? Did she need a new little girl to love? We were best friends. Why did she need a baby, too?

"I'm going to my room," was all I said.

Other kids might've had a fascination with the progress of the pregnancy, but I worked hard at blocking it out. I kept my eyes on Mom's face and tried to let the rest of her body float unfocused at the edge of my vision. If I didn't see it, it didn't exist. I lined up as much babysitting as I could to get out of the house, and I started studying in my room instead of the kitchen so I didn't have to catch any unwanted glimpses of her. After a while, though, there was no denying that belly.

Mom did her best to win me over. "If you don't pick anything crazy, you can name the baby," she told me. I know she wanted me to start bonding with this thing I'd reviled, and I was grudgingly moving toward not hating it. One saving grace was that it was a boy—and a boy couldn't possibly have the same relationship with Mom that I had. I settled on the name Christopher. Emmett's last name was Carmen, and Christopher Carmen had a ring to it. I thought it sounded catchy, like Kris Kringle.

Mom and Emmett waited until almost the end of the school year to drop their final bomb. We were moving. And this time it wasn't just across the floating bridge. Mom had gotten a dream job in San Diego, and there was nothing to say to the opportunity but yes. After dogpaddling through the bureaucracy for years, Mom had finally wound up with bosses and mentors who saw her potential. They were naming her director of the San Diego field office of the EEOC.

I understood why we had to do it, and how much it would do to put our struggles behind us. But what if our life changed too much? New city, new school, new baby, Emmett. I was the only "old" thing left.

I finished up at Lakeside carried more by momentum than anything resembling concentration. For once I had no idea where I stood in my class, and grades were the last thing on my mind. My final weeks there were a long good-bye. With nothing to lose, I finally summoned the courage to tell a boy I'd watched from afar for three years that I liked him. It didn't go well. He just looked at me like I was completely clueless and said, "Oh. I thought you knew I like someone else." Suddenly moving didn't seem like such a bad idea.

My hardest good-bye was with Paige. I thought about what to give her to remember me by, and since she already had everything she could want, I decided to wrap up something that was one of a kind. It was a collage of images, mostly torn from magazines, that I thought were beautiful. Movie stars, singers, models, magazine photos of Paris and other places I'd never seen: Every time I was struck by a face or a mood or the color of a dress, I'd cut out an image and add it to the collage. It had hung on the back of my bedroom door through many moves, and I could lie in bed and look at it, dreaming myself into places and bodies and futures that felt less like a fantasy than a taste of what my life could be.

I could tell Paige didn't know what to say when she unwrapped it. Instead of looking at it and asking me about it, the way I'd imagined she would, she put it down on her bed with a quick "Wow, thanks, Lisa" and changed the subject by saying, "I have something for you, too." I recognized the look on her face. It was the same embarrassed smile I'd gotten when I brought my paper dollhouse to school in fourth grade. When I looked at the collage through her eyes, it was just a collection of sad scraps. Trash. I'd been fooling myself. Maybe it really was time to move on.

EIGHT

A Trapdoor into Medicine

Christopher announced himself with a flourish as Mom and I were visiting one of the best schools in metro San Diego.

The Bishop's School, just a few blocks from the beach, had the feel of a college campus, with Spanish-style buildings arranged around a huge, grassy courtyard and a bell tower with a carillon that marked the hours. The whole air of the place seemed familiar, with kids in uniforms not so different from the ones we'd worn at Epiphany and a chapel at one end of the quad. Bishop's roots were Episcopal, and it had only recently become coed after years as a girls' school. I'd missed the admissions cutoff for the coming year, but I could secure my spot in the tenth grade class by going in during the summer to take the entrance exam. I wasn't worried about passing it, but I was anxious about making another good impression. It was never easy to be new again.

Test day arrived at the end of June, and Mom and I were climbing the wide stairs to the main office when I heard a whooshing sound and saw a flood of liquid rushing down Mom's leg. Her water had broken. Christopher was supposed to be a "by appointment" C-section baby, but he obviously had other plans.

"Mom!" I said, scared and horrified. "What's wrong? What happened?"

"Let's just get to the front desk," she said. "I'm going to have the baby."

She stood outside the door for a moment so the fluid could drain away and she'd drip less in the hallway, then she calmly marched me to the desk.

"My daughter is here to take the test," she told the secretaries. "I have to go to the hospital. I'll try to arrange for someone to pick her up, but please take care of her till someone can come."

The secretaries fluttered nervously, offering to call someone who could drive her, and I pleaded with Mom to sit down. But she straightened herself up, said she'd be okay, and walked back to her car.

There was nothing for me to do but go in and take the test.

My mind worked word puzzles and solved equations on autopilot while I fretted about Mom. I didn't know if I was doing well or badly, but I kept flipping pages until there were no more questions. The secretaries had called to check on Mom, and when I got out they said she'd made it to the delivery room and she was doing fine. They found books for me to read and hovered with snacks and murmured reassurances until Emmett showed up to take me to see her. She was already resting with the baby in her arms. I had to hand it to Christopher: He'd managed not to keep her in labor for hours—and he was kind of cute. I hadn't expected him to be so small.

I wish I could say that it was the first sight of my baby brother that made me realize I wanted to devote my life to infants and their mothers. But it was nothing like that. Mom's return home with Christopher marked the beginning of the worst summer of my life. Mom had her new job to attend to, and in just two weeks she was back at the office full time, trying to learn the ropes while making her mark as the new boss. Emmett was home from the Panama Canal for another couple of weeks, but he had to work when he was in port. That left me alone with a newborn from the time Mom left in the morning until she returned at 5:30 or 6. I think she was assuming that little Christopher would simply sleep for most of that time, but he was an active, fussy baby with a good pair of lungs. I was in over my head.

What I remember most about that summer is how dark and closed-in our apartment was. Mom and Emmett hadn't had much time to look, and we'd landed temporarily in a cramped and cave-like first-floor unit that was worse than even the "motel" Mom and I had lived in at our low point in Seattle. It was next to a noisy stair-well, and there wasn't a glimmer of natural light. When everyone was home, we were on top of each other.

Mom showed me how to prepare the baby's formula and change his diapers, and all day every day I stayed indoors trying to keep him from crying—because once he started, practically nothing would make him stop.

I have one strong word of caution for moms today: Don't even think about putting your newborn in the full-time care of a thirteen-year-old girl, no matter how mature you believe she is. Case in point: me at my worst. I was so frustrated in the midst of one of Christopher's colicky bouts of despair that I called my mother's office and insisted on being put through.

"If you don't come get this baby right now, I'm going to put him in the trash," I told Mom, much to her horror.

"You will do no such thing," she yelled. "Go get him right now. Where is he? In his crib? How could you say such a thing! Don't you dare hurt that child!"

"I wasn't really gonna do it, but the thing was driving me crazy," I backpedaled. "I wasn't cut out for this."

"I'll be home in a few hours," she said. "I want you to call me at three and at four, do you understand, and tell me how he is. How could you even think of saying something like that?"

When she got home that night, I brought the baby to her and said, "See, he's fine. You take him." Then I did what I'd do every evening until I went back to school: I shoved my new brother into her arms, got on my bike, and rode as far away as I could, staying out until dark. It would be my turn to take care of the baby again in the middle of the night. Mom couldn't afford to go in to work in that new-mother state of sleep-deprived spaciness, so I was in charge of preparing his bottles and getting up to feed him. He woke me every few hours.

On one of my long evening bike rides, I spotted my salvation: a bright yellow flyer on a telephone pole. It was an ad seeking candy stripers for the local hospital. I'd never been interested in hospitals or medicine—I was more the detective type, I thought—but when I saw the ad, wheels began to turn. They wanted volunteers who could come in on weekends and after school, and if I worked things right, I might be able to fill up a lot of my free time, a.k.a. my baby-sitting hours, with this when school started again. If the choice was between being with sick people and spending more time with the little screamer, it was no contest. My mom would probably go for it, because who could argue with medicine? It sounded serious and academic.

I tore down the flyer, tucked it into my pocket and called the number the next day. I was right about Mom. When the information sheets arrived and I told her I was thinking about medicine as a career since I liked science, she signed me up.

I needn't have worried about staying busy. September brought a rush of activity when classes started at Francis Parker, the high school I'd be attending until I could go to Bishop's. Parker was another top-tier school, with a modern campus and a friendly, down-to-earth atmosphere. It had some of the rigor I was used to, but after my long months of servitude in our dungeon of a house, everything felt easy to me, almost like a vacation. I was relaxed and happy at Parker, and I thrived. Parker wasn't as hard as Lakeside, and it didn't take much to stay ahead.

I dreamed up one ambitious project with my uncle Don, who visited us in San Diego when his ship came in. For my math class we were supposed to create something three-dimensional that had geometric symmetry, and Don, an engineer, came up with the idea of building the Taj Mahal from sugar cubes. He still remembers how I pestered him about it and how once we got going, it was "sugar cubes and superglue for days." He also remembers the way I called him when I got an A minus on our dazzling creation, while other kids got As for simpler projects. Completely forgoing any thanks, I complained: "We could've done a mobile!" Still, I'd come a long, long way from the paper dollhouse.

I tried out for cheerleader and made the squad, landed leading roles in the school plays, and sang solos in the musicals. As usual I was at the top of my class, but this time I was also one of the popular kids.

With all my rehearsals and meetings, I could've dropped the idea of volunteering at the hospital, but the training sessions were on Saturdays, and going would all but rule out another round of child-care duty. I liked the uniforms, too.

I hoped the tasks they gave me would be exciting. Mostly, though, they were mundane, especially at the beginning. A good part of our training was an orientation to the hospital, with emphasis on places where we'd be spending a lot of time, such as the various lab and waiting areas and the delivery room, where we'd pick up flowers, magazines, and newspapers to shuttle to patients' rooms. Rule No. 1 was: The nurse is God—do what she says. I learned to file, make beds, handle medical wastes safely, deliver blood and urine samples or X-rays to the lab, and pick up results. And then I waited for a spot to open up on the regular candy-striper roster. I finally got a placement in the spring.

As all candy stripers have for eons, we wore red-and-white-striped jumpers over white blouses, a uniform that made us stand out from the medical staff and the patients or visitors. I was content with that semioutsider status and satisfied just to be getting out of the house. But bit by bit, the hospital began to seduce me. One afternoon I was sent to the rehabilitation wards to deliver some newspapers and found myself face to face with Desi Arnaz Jr., son of Lucy and Desi, and his girlfriend Linda Purl, who'd starred in *Happy Days*. They were a high-wattage couple at the time, and that first star meeting (I managed a semicalm "Hi, how are you?") gave the hospital a sheen of glamour.

Soon, though, I discovered something far more intoxicating—the feeling that I could be of use when it really counted. Once I'd become a fixture around the wards, a busy nurse stopped me and asked if I could help feed a patient. "The man in there can't lift his hands," she told me, pointing to a dim doorway, "so he needs help eating."

What she didn't mention was that the same accident that had cost the man his hands had also devastated his head, seeming to melt away his features. "He just has half a face," my mind repeated as I tried to look into his good eye, lifting the spoon again and again to the irregular line of his mouth. I was struck by how hard he had to work simply to take in food and how much he needed me.

When he was finished, I found the nurse. "You probably should've warned me about the man's face. Some people would freak out," I told her, tacitly indicating that I hadn't.

"God, I didn't even think about it," she said. It was second nature to the nurses simply to do what needed to be done—there wasn't time or energy for shock. I understood that now—I felt it, and it surprised me. I didn't want to run away from the man. I wanted to do more to help him.

I saw that part of myself again one day as I waited for my mom to pick me up after school. A young boy had fallen off some equipment on the playground, and teachers had brought him into the headmaster's room near where I sat. The boy's arm was bent in the wrong direction, clearly broken, and he was in so much pain he was sweating. He screamed and cried. The secretary ran around, trying to call his mother and decide if we needed an ambulance. "See if you can calm him down," she yelled in my direction.

I sat next to the boy and grabbed his hand. "It's going to be okay. Your mom will come get you," I repeated. And then I started telling him stories to see if I could make him laugh. Jokes, anything I could think of. The raw howls thinned to hiccups of sobs, and sooner than I could've expected, the crying had stopped. I kept talking and clinging to the boy's hand until his mom arrived.

I kept an eye out for him in the weeks after that, and when I finally saw him again, his arm was wrapped in a long white cast, and his face had a five-hundred-watt smile for me. He handed me a thank-you note and gave me a one-armed hug. I didn't know exactly how I'd found a way to comfort him—maybe it came from soothing Mom on her bad days. And I was sure I had it in me to do it again for someone else. Pain and blood didn't scare me. I could find my way to the eye of the storm, gather myself and know what was needed. I saw that about myself now.

Our home life was a peaceful backdrop for a while. Our second place in San Diego had a pool, and when I wasn't at rehearsals or the hospital, I'd do my homework out on the deck and swim till I was exhausted. I lost a lot of my baby fat doing that and started to feel less like the awkward briefcase girl from Seattle and more like the California cheerleader I'd become.

When Emmett wanted to be closer to the water, we moved to Solana Beach, a small town about twenty miles north of San Diego. He and Mom had been married for about a year, and for the most part things seemed to be working—especially with his work taking him away from us for long stretches. Any tension seemed to dissolve when he left, and his homecomings were full of excitement for Christopher and Mom. My instincts about him were confirmed, though, when I overheard one of his telephone conversations.

"Controlling old bitch," he was telling someone. I knew he was talking about Mom. "She's always on me. Damn! And that girl of hers. . . ." He went on like that, talking about how she just wanted the baby, not him.

I knew there was truth in that, but I was incensed. It probably wasn't possible for me to mistrust him more than I already did, but now that I knew how he really felt about Mom, I couldn't pretend I didn't know what he was up to. Fortunately, his stays at home were getting shorter and shorter.

There was one other huge change during that first stretch of our California life. After Emmett went back out to sea and we were alone again, Mom skidded into a depression about her luck with men and her post-Christopher body, which showed signs of sagging just the way my grandmother's did. I did something to irritate her—it probably involved asking at the last minute for yet another ride to an after-school function—and her smoldering mood flamed.

"Get the belt," she said.

I hesitated.

"Get the damn belt!"

I pulled it out of the closet and handed it to her. By now I didn't know what was worse: the pain of the strap or the mortification of stripping in front of her. I was starting to go through puberty, and the embarrassment was more than I could bear. As I stepped out of my clothes, I tried to arrange my arms so they'd cover me. It was such a laughable effort that I had to just let them fall. I couldn't do this anymore.

I turned around slowly.

"No, Mom. Don't, please don't," I said, looking her in the eye. "This isn't right, Mommy. We're so close, and you're still using the belt on me. You wouldn't do that to anyone else, Mom. Don't hit me."

I don't know why I felt calm, but I did. Mom stood frozen in front of me, but she couldn't hold my gaze. I knew it was over when she slumped to the bed and started to cry.

I picked up my clothes and started to dress. She saw something new in me, I think. Or maybe she finally saw what she was doing. She'd get irritated once in a while and slap me across the face, but she never hit me with the belt again.

Nine

Haynesville

Haynesville, Louisiana, sits just a few miles from the Arkansas border, surrounded by pinewoods, red oak, and hickory. I went back for summer stays all my life, settling—at least for a week or two—into the slow pace of life in the small Southern town where my mom grew up. Haynesville was my "what if": What if Mom had never left? What if we'd stayed entwined in our roots? I know Mom sent me there to let me feel part of a large family with layers of history. But those trips were also a way of saying, "See? You're bigger than my past. That world was too small for you and me."

It was a tiny place. A steady two thousand people or so lived in the area, though the population had swelled briefly to twenty thousand in the 1920s when an oil strike turned Haynesville into a boomtown. There had always been about as many whites as blacks living there, though even in post–civil rights days they didn't mix much. The WPA mural in the post office showed heroic-looking white farmers near their barns and a separate vignette of heroic-looking black men and women who lugged huge sacks of cotton.

That scraped-from-the-soil life was our history. My grandmother, Mattie Ruth Smith, had helped pick cotton when she was young, one of eleven children in a close farm family. Her father was a carpenter and a minister, and five of his girls became teachers. Grandma tried a few other jobs—receptionist for a doctor, worker in a government program for children—but once she'd set her mind on teaching, she went for a degree at the Louisiana Negro Normal and Industrial Institute, which would become Grambling State University. She taught at black schools during the academic year and spent her summers on her college work, doggedly earning her degree. She was twenty-three when her father died, and she stepped into the void, taking on the task of being sure the cows were milked, the fields plowed, and the business of the farm tended to, along with her five younger siblings, who were still at home.

Grandma's three older sisters were teaching in other towns, and her elder brothers were either teaching or in the military, all of them sending money home to help the family. Grandma was happy to be in charge. "She was like a little mother to us," remembers my Aunt Geneva, who was ten years younger. "She kept the farm running—whatever there was to do, she made sure we did it." Geneva says Grandma was a commanding personality who always had to have the last word on everything. "She was just bossy," Geneva says.

I remember that side of her as well, but I also saw that, at least where I was concerned, discipline and directives were always delivered with a twinkle in the eye. Below her tough exterior was a big heart, and I knew she had a soft spot for me.

Grandma fell in love with a tall, handsome farmer named Roy Smith, and she was twenty-five and pregnant when he went off to join Gen. George S. Patton's Third Army in France after the invasion of Normandy. He was gone for four years and sent home every penny he earned, the story went, except what he spent on toothpaste and tobacco. His salary became their nest egg—Grandma saved it all and provided for Mom and herself on her teacher's salary.

She was essentially a single mom for the first years of my mother's life. The two of them were a lot like Mom and me: inseparable. Grandma took her new daughter everywhere with her, and by age three Mom was perched in the back of a classroom with the big kids, absorbing their lessons. The intense bond that developed between Mom and Grandma then was there for a lifetime and so was Mom's devotion to education. Having gotten a huge push at the beginning, she had gut-level knowledge of how much a tiny child is capable of learning when there's more than kindergarten fare on offer.

Mom didn't recognize Grandpa when he finally came home, and she howled for days at being displaced from her mother's bed. After that rocky reentry Grandma and Grandpa took their time readjusting to family life and the rhythms of peacetime. They were a pious couple who'd spend all day Sunday at church, with Grandma singing and playing piano for choirs in all the nearby towns. Mom remained an only child for a couple of more years, and she was six when my uncle Don was born. My uncle Almer came along a couple of years later. Mom always described the boys as a mischievous pair, and she often told the story of how Don made off with her earrings and attached them to the unwitting cat or tied bells to it. But as happens in families, Don tells a slightly different story.

"I distinctly remember the cat coming in with bells," he says, "and I don't remember a thing about having anything to do with it. La V'onne stuck to that story to the very end, but she was the one with the mischief, and she could always manipulate the facts. I think she had a tremendous desire for attention after Dad came home; then I came along. She felt like she was getting robbed, and Mother didn't have the skills to make her feel secure."

Mom's most notorious prank was persuading little Almer that he could fly and daring him to jump off the roof wearing the "magic cape" she made him. (He came away with a broken arm, and she had hell to pay.) Disturbing as that story was, I could identify with what was behind it. I hadn't had the easiest time getting used to my brother Christopher, after all. Not after the intensity of being alone with Mom for so long. I could feel history flowing into a familiar groove.

When Mom got old enough to date, it irritated her to no end that she had to be chaperoned by one of the boys. In keeping with an Old South tradition, the brothers stayed in the room when her suitors came to call, and there were plenty of suitors for a fair-skinned, good-looking young woman.

My uncles remember the way Mom let nothing—not them, not their girlfriends, not anyone—come between her and her mother's attentions. Ever. She went off to college at Grambling at sixteen and got her start teaching in the nearby town of Coushatta, then in Shreveport, the nearest city, seventy miles away. And practically every day for the rest of her life, she called home to stay close to Grandma.

I imagine that the farm I experienced on my summer visits was still much like the one Mom had known. The four-room, two-porch house Grandma and Grandpa had started out with had been added to as the family had grown, and it stretched out comfortably behind the large oak that shaded the front yard and carport.

The front door now opened into a large room with Grandma and Grandpa's bed and sofas, a sort of bedroom/sitting room, so we generally used the side door right off the carport, going through the formal living room and dining room to a long, cool hallway that became a refuge from the heat when my cousin Angie and I closed it off and turned up the air-conditioning, lounging on a sofa and reading magazines. Several bedrooms, including one that had been kept exactly as Mom had left it, opened off the hall.

The back of the house was its heart. The kitchen faced Grandpa's acres of fields, and next to it were the laundry room and the study, where a whole collection of diplomas, and photos of the family's proud college graduates, lined the walls. In a stereotypical

Southern town where opportunities for blacks were few and far between, and most professions were closed to them, nearly every one of Grandma's siblings had gone to Grambling and gotten a teaching degree.

My grandmother's books filled shelf after shelf. Shakespeare, classics such as the *Iliad* and the *Odyssey* that I'd encountered at school, the Bible, Plato. Philosophy, literature. I would lose myself in the stories, the third generation of the Smith women to take refuge and find a future in those well-dusted volumes, cherished since Grandma's college days. It must've been in our DNA to love them.

Much as I could've spent all my time holed up inside with books and magazines, there was no getting around the fact that this was still a working farm. I may have been a night owl, but the roosters didn't care. Their riotous noise set the day in motion mid-dream, with the sound of my grandfather's heavy boots and the slap of the screen door signaling the start of his long hours of tending cows and crops. He had eighty acres of cotton, corn, peanuts, and hay and an array of cattle, pigs, chickens, and turkeys to care for. Soon Grandma would be at the stove preparing a huge breakfast of eggs and sausage and grits for him (and us) to eat when he came back in. She sent me once to the henhouse out back to fetch eggs from the nests, but the chickens scared me with their intense tiny eyes; sharp, exposed edges; and unpredictable flapping. I refused to go back into the dank, squawking dark.

I was no match, either, for the cattle that roamed the fields. I wanted to look at them up close, but having been warned to stay away from the temperamental bulls, I thought it best to avoid anything remotely bovine. I didn't know how to tell bulls from cows. I couldn't even fish. It looked idyllic when Grandpa sat on the banks of the pond he'd long ago carved into a field, but when he took me out for the first time, I starred in another "can't take the city out of the girl" episode. I caught a fish, much to my delight, but I

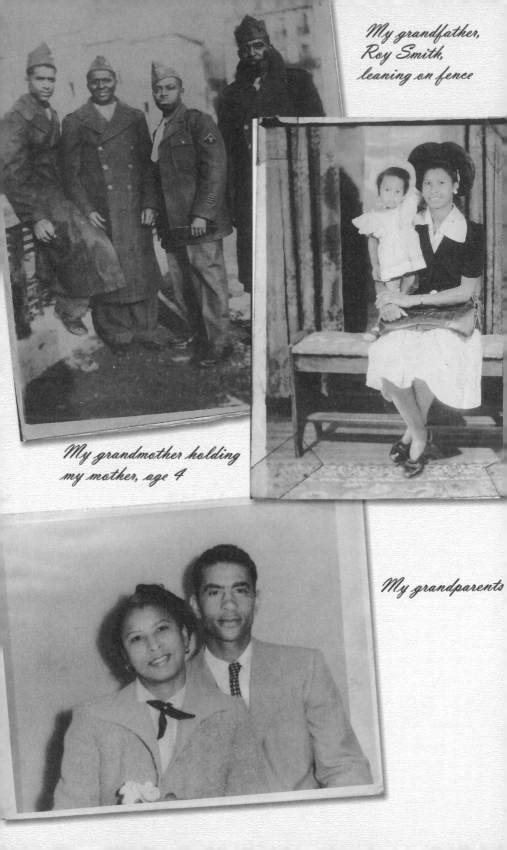

My grandfather,
Roy Smith,
leaning on fence

My grandmother holding
my mother, age 4

My grandparents

somehow managed to lodge a hook in my hand. That traumatized both Grandpa and me so badly that I didn't pick up a pole again until many years later, when fly-fishing sounded romantic enough to get me into waders. Grandpa stopped mentioning fishing when I was around.

Passing a part of the summer in the South meant contending with flies, mosquitoes, and air so thick and hot that it seemed to melt over your skin and weigh you down—it was no wonder people moved so slowly. My encounters with extreme nature always left me exhausted for the first few days. But it didn't matter. Grandma was determined to weave me into the fabric of the farm and the larger family, and I was fully booked.

Angie, who was a couple of years younger than I, was my uncle Don's daughter and my most constant playmate. She was light-skinned where I was dark, and her hair was "better" than mine, longer and a lot less nappy. She was also tall and thin, whereas I was short and plump, so she didn't get lectures from Grandma about losing weight. But then, she didn't get the doting that came with being the first grandchild, either. We were rivals, and we jostled for our grandparents' attention—I believed I was entitled to them since she could see them anytime—but we both liked to roller-skate, and between that, riding bikes, and making mud houses in the red dirt under the front-yard tree, we could generally amuse ourselves.

Grandma, of course, had plans for us as well. That bossiness my aunt Geneva grumbled about was on full display as my grand-mother put us to work doing dishes or dusting or helping her can the mountains of apples and pears from the orchards next to the house. There was weeding in the garden, chicken feed to scatter, fat round peas to push from their shells, corn to shuck. All day Sunday, Grandma and Grandpa were in church, which meant fidgeting through the preaching, joining in with the singing, and finally being excused to run outside when it was clear Angie and I couldn't stifle our giggles a moment longer.

Mom generally flew down to Haynesville with me, staying just a couple of days before she went home. I loved to see her relax and laugh with family and old friends. "Baby Rae," they called her. "See, my phone's not ringing," Grandma would say in the afternoon, the time Mom usually called her to check in. A stream of relatives dropped by the house, and we made a circuit as well. I drank oceans of grape and orange soda.

Grandma did her best to ensure that I saw my dad, who had remarried and lived nearby with his new wife and her family. I was never eager to do it—he was someone else's daddy now—but in Grandma's eyes a father was a father. I could see traces of my face in his.

Haynesville was by turns idyllic (summer on a farm!), boring ("Grandma, I can't find anything to do; I'm going to bed now"), and eye-opening. Perhaps most difficult for me as I got older was seeing how my grandmother, so take-charge and assertive in the church and family, deferred to the white folks in town. Before a trip to the Piggly Wiggly, she'd urge me to mind my manners and "just smile and make nice." But I was my mother's daughter, and back home Mom was a force to be reckoned with when she perceived a slight, demanding to talk to the restaurant manager when we were seated near the kitchen. She didn't do "don't make waves"—she preferred to swamp the ship of anyone she thought had treated us with anything less than respect.

When my brother Christopher was two, I got my clearest sense of why Mom couldn't have survived the small-town South. He became feverish early in our stay, and Grandma packed us up and drove us to the doctor's office in town, steering us to the blacks-only entrance around back.

"Grandma, we can't go in here. Let's go in the other side, in the front," I told her, refusing to move. I held Christopher in my arms. He was heavy and very hot. But I didn't budge.

"Lisa, you want Christopher to get better, don't you? Don't argue with me. We need to get him inside. Stop making a fuss." She pushed the door open to reveal a bare, whitewashed room with a linoleum floor and a few worn chairs. It was stark, utilitarian, and unlike any doctor's office I'd ever seen. As soon as the nurse took my grandmother and Christopher through a door and into an exam room, I ran around to the front of the building to get a look at what was behind the "white" door.

It was an ordinary waiting room, but it was plush by comparison, with carpeting, upholstered chairs, a coffee table with well-thumbed magazines, and a counter with a frosted pane of glass that slid open to reveal the startled face of the receptionist.

"You should be ashamed of yourself," I told her, my heart pounding so loudly I was sure she could hear it. "Why can't my brother come in here? He's just as good as anyone else." I was used to annoying questions from people about my hair, and I knew how to think about the guys who didn't consider me girlfriend material because of my color. They were kids, stupid kids. But this was a doctor's office, and doctors were supposed to treat everyone the same, not look at someone's color before they decided who got the best treatment. My mom wouldn't stand for it. They had no right.

I did my best to slam the door on the way out and went back to the other side to wait for my grandmother and Christopher. How could she trust a doctor who'd do this? I could feel my anger sizzling into tears.

"I saw the other office," I blurted out when she emerged. Her face tightened, and I thought she was going to slap me, but instead she just said, "Let's go outside." I took Christopher, and she held onto the white square of a prescription form.

Out on the sidewalk she looked more sad than angry. "Honey, you all are going to leave soon, but your Grandpa and I have to stay here, and it will be very difficult for me if you ever do anything like that again. You can't just come in and change everything all at once."

I didn't believe her. I still don't. The image of that bare, run-down waiting room that was "the way things have always been" in Haynesville has never left me.

In the years since that time, I've been inspired to hear about how my Grandpa coped with segregation and the battles to end it. He and my uncles were often shut out of the tightly closed circle my mom and grandma made—the matriarchy, as my uncles refer to it—so his story wasn't one of the ones they told and retold. But it turned out that Grandpa was the one who'd stood up to protect the black freedom marchers in town, a "deacon of defense" in the Masons who took it as an extension of his post to see that the marchers came to no harm. Grandma wouldn't participate because she was afraid of losing her job, but Grandpa put himself on the line. The truth was a little larger, a little more complicated, than what I'd been able to see looking through Mom's and Grandma's eyes. Mom, and maybe I, just might've gotten our spark from him.

TEN

Love

I was in my element when I finally arrived at Bishop's. Everything about it fit—the sea of uniforms, the feeling of history in the classrooms, and traditions like "M&C," milk and cookies time, which brought the whole school together on the patio at ten every morning for refreshments. I was well familiar with the campus because we'd been attending St. James Church, right next door, since we moved to San Diego. The congregation welcomed us warmly, and I was invited to be an altar girl. St. James was fine with having a black girl lighting candles and helping priests prepare for rituals, a dot of color among the predominately white—and male—acolytes. The church made me feel embraced by community the way I wanted to be in Haynesville.

After services on Sundays I'd walk around the Bishop's campus, imagining myself as a student, and it felt like home by the time I was ready to join the tenth-grade class. The school was an intimate place, with its classes of eight to ten and a cozy library warmed by a fireplace. I was still one of the only black students on campus, but fresh from my "popular girl" year at Parker, I was poised to fit in. Especially with new contact lenses and my first trip to the salon for a relaxer. Wearing my hair down, and free of my heavy glasses, I could finally shed the last vestiges of my nerdy-girl skin. These were my swan years.

I made friends as I always had, finding them as I waited for my mom to pick me up after school. She worked in a fancy downtown office with an expansive view of the harbor, and she reveled in running her own show. But it was harder than ever for her to get away at the end of the day, and I had to amuse myself for hours until she did. As the afternoons wore on, the only people left on campus were the boarders who lived in the dorm. One of them, Christina, was a slender girl of Indian descent who had long black hair, thick, wavy, and hippie style. She hung out on the steps after hours, and soon we were fast friends. Her family lived in Arizona, and they didn't seem rich, so I got the idea that they were doing what Mom and I had done—making sure she got a good education that they couldn't necessarily afford. Christina didn't talk about them much, and she didn't seem to miss them, either.

I think she was the one who pointed out the three Marks, a trio of guys who were always walking past on the way to Baskin-Robbins. Mark Sansone was a surfer kid with long, dirty blond hair, Vans sneakers, and a quiet way about him. Mark Stang was a short, witty, brainiac with glasses who liked to trade quips with me. And Marc Wintress was a tall, artsy type who was on the sensitive side. I had a crush on the surfer. The Marks were in all my classes, and before too long they started including me in homework sessions in the library and gossip on the steps. We'd walk around the school or to the beach, talking. I liked being one of the guys, and I kept my crush to myself when it looked as though I was the only one thinking "couple."

In solidarity with our little gang, I volunteered to manage the baseball team they were all on—a job that basically involved keeping score, not devising strategy. I might well have joined the team if they'd let girls play. I would've been happy if any one of the Marks could've liked me in a more romantic way, but it wasn't to be, probably, I thought, because I wasn't attractive enough.

I was determined to make up for that with smarts and personality. I became a cheerleader (which at Bishop's had more to do with rousing school spirit than boosting a sports team), performed with a group called the Madrigals that sang at private schools up and down the coast, tutored disadvantaged kids in reading and math after school, and continued with my candy striping. I was probably too busy to date.

By now Emmett had completely faded from our lives. I hardly realized it had happened at first. He kept sending checks, but the long stretches between visits finally connected into one long absence, and he simply disappeared. There was no trauma, and just as I don't remember a wedding, I don't remember a divorce. It was just a gradual sputtering out. In the end, though, everyone came away with what they wanted: Mom had Christopher, Emmett had his freedom, and I had Mom back.

Mom and I thrived during that first year at Bishop's. We were living within our means in a small condo in La Costa, twenty miles north of the school's pricey La Jolla neighborhood, the same approach we'd used in Seattle—favoring the cheaper suburbs. Emmett's checks were regular, Mom had reached a career peak, I was on scholarship with college in my future, and Christopher was there for Mom to love when I was gone. Romance was the only thing missing from the picture, and Mom was so taken up with her job and minding a toddler that she didn't seem to care.

I was the one who needed to fall in love, and I did, more than once.

The first time it happened I was at the hospital. A nurse sent me to the emergency room on an errand, and I stood there swallowed up by the chaos. The doctors and nurses rushed around me with an intensity that made me calm. These were people who would focus their last ounce of energy on you when you came through their doors, doing everything they could to save your life or make you feel better. I wanted to soak up that feeling, and I lingered much longer than I was supposed to. All around me I could feel the same extreme need I'd seen in the man with half a face—and it pulled me in.

I dropped in to see the woman in charge of the candy stripers' program and gave her my best pitch. "I think I want to be a doctor," I told her. "I'm taking science classes at Bishop's, and I want to be in the ER. I'll do anything you want if I can be assigned there."

A lot of discussion ensued on the hospital staff about whether it made sense to let me volunteer there, much of it some variation on the theme: "The emergency room is no place for kids."

"We haven't had anyone as young as you in the ER," the volunteer coordinator told me. "It could be overwhelming for you, and that wouldn't be good for anyone."

"What if I just observe and stay out of the way," I countered. She told me they'd think about it.

At last, with warnings that there was no telling what I'd see, and that some of it would probably be traumatic, I got the okay to be there for a regular eight-hour shift on Saturdays. If I wanted immersion, there it was. I would be the charge of a young orderly named Roger.

Roger was happy to have me. The low man on the totem pole now had someone a notch lower to supervise. I helped him wheel gurneys from place to place and set up surgical trays, and I watched as he navigated among the professional staff and the patients, making jokes and asking questions. He was in his early twenties and preparing to apply to medical school, so he got as close to the doctors and nurses as he could, hoping for recommendations. In turn they let him sew up wounds and learn basics that were beyond his job description. I was the apprentice's apprentice, doing his bidding and free to observe any procedures I wanted to see. I was fascinated by chest tubes. But then, I was fascinated by everything. The more I saw, the more certain I was that I really did want to be a doctor. I was smitten.

Mom liked my new career direction, but she wasn't thrilled by the driving involved in my volunteer work. "Why do you have to help all those people," she complained. "I don't have time for this." She was stretched thin. Christopher was a more scattered child than I'd been, and he was beginning to need more attention. Mom's job was in overdrive as well. She was great at talking her way into a position, but once she arrived she found that people wanted her to deliver on all the promise in her résumé. If there was a façade involved—and often in Mom's life there was—it took a lot of energy to maintain it. She came home often talking about having to watch her back and fend off people who wanted her to fail. She also had stories of working with people like Clarence Thomas, before he was a household name. She didn't have a lot left for my transportation needs.

That's how I wound up driving alone at age fifteen and a half, ferrying myself to the hospital or running errands for Mom. Grandpa had taught me to drive his big pink Cadillac on the quiet roads around the farm when I was too short to see over the dashboard, propping me up on phone books and pushing the seat up as far as it would go so I could reach the pedals. I'd done all right with that, so once I got my learner's permit in San Diego, Mom dispensed with the "adult must be present" rule and let me drive short distances from the house without her. She'd accompany me on the first run to a new destination, and when she was content that I could handle the route, I was on my own. "Your whole future will go right out the window if you hit someone," she cautioned, "so be careful."

I checked my mirrors obsessively for police and stayed within the speed limit, especially since I suspected we didn't have car insurance. The longer Emmett was gone, the more I could feel us sliding back to our familiar shaky ground. Day care was expensive, and there was always some incidental cost at my school: a new costume, a class trip, materials for a project. We began to juggle again. And even at that there were things that remained out of reach. I longed to go with the art history group from my school that toured Europe every year, but that would have to wait.

Church was a haven. I continued as an acolyte on Sundays and began attending at wedding services. I spent even more time at St. James after the bishop took a liking to me and asked me to be his personal altar girl, which meant helping prepare for additional services, particularly around the high holy days. I never lost the sense of awe I felt in the midst of the rituals, and I enjoyed the kids involved in the church's youth group, which, beyond its liberal mix of such activities as camping trips, movie and pizza nights, and car washes, occasionally ventured into the realm of serious spirituality. Mom sent me to a weekend retreat led by the priests where cautionary messages about respecting yourself by waiting to have sex and stories about the transformative power of caring for other people built to a larger message that came together on the last day, when each of us was given a bag that contained notes from the people who cared about us the most. My mother and grandmother both wrote about how much I meant to them, and though they'd never been shy about letting me know, when I saw their words, Grandma's in her perfect teacher's handwriting, I felt wrapped up in love. I knew the whole exercise was engineered to do that, but I couldn't discount how good it felt.

I was sixteen and participating in a service at St. James when a transfer student named Tom Darby walked down the aisle. At a priest's cue he began to recite something in flawless French. I stared. He had a mischievous Tom Sawyer quality about him, with freckles, reddish dirty brown hair, hazel eyes, and a broad smile. And that French! I made a point of introducing myself.

When I found out that his accent came courtesy of his family's recent stay in France, where his father had been posted in the military, I quizzed him about Europe, practiced my French on him, and began seeking him out after school, walking to the beach, talking. Tom was two grades below me and a year younger, and I didn't read much into the time we were spending together. I volunteered to manage the basketball team (more stats and scorekeeping) so I could be with him the same way I was with the Marks—as the girl who's the friend but not the girlfriend.

So it shocked me when Tom took my hand one day as we walked on the campus. My whole body responded to that touch, the long, slender fingers of a fresh-faced fifteen-year-old slipping between mine and somehow weaving us together. It was as purely erotic as anything I've ever felt. It seemed that the next best thing to going to Paris, which had been my dream practically since my first French lesson in grade school, was to fall for a cosmopolitan boy who'd lived there.

Tom gave me my first kiss, just a simple, dry meeting of lips, during another walk that spring. I glowed with it, but it was nothing compared with our first contact. I wasn't in a position to say kissing was overrated, but I didn't quite get what the fuss was about until we tried it again during finals week. Tom found me early in the day and told me to meet him in the prayer garden behind the chapel before my English test. The garden, with its tumbling bougainvilleas and the sweet perfume of honeysuckle and roses, was a popular destination not only for contemplation but also for making out. Tom led me to a secluded corner and said, "Now I'm going to teach you how to really kiss. Do what I do. You'll like it better."

His mouth seemed softer than before, and his tongue made me aware of the endless smoothness of our lips. This was a new kind of contact, breath to breath. My head was spinning, and I sank to the ground. Tom sat down with me, and the kiss went on until I heard bells—literal ones to mark the end of the class period.

I raced into my final flustered and did my best to pull myself from the garden scene still playing behind my eyes. I wasn't sure how I answered the questions, and I wrote a note on the last page of the test that read:

"Sorry if I was distracted. I just got my first kiss, and I'm so dizzy I can't concentrate."

I was glad to announce that the long drought was over.

Tom and I went out after his ball games and paired up for movies, but our nascent dating life ran into resistance from his mother, who called Mom and asked her to keep us apart. The reason? I was black, and that was "not something she wanted for her son." The poor woman had no idea whom she was talking to.

"And you're saying my daughter isn't good enough for him? Is that what you're telling me?" Mom said. "I can't even dignify that with a response." The receiver went down hard. She swore under her breath.

"He's a great kid, Leese," she told me, "unlike his mother. You two do whatever you want to—I'm glad to see you happy."

Tom told his parents he'd stop seeing me, but we continued to meet, with forays into the prayer garden. Our dating would only be a problem if his parents came to a basketball game and saw us together there—which, of course, they did. They didn't make a scene at the time, but they yanked him out of Bishop's and sent him across town to La Jolla High. We tried to stay connected over the summer, but by the time school started again, the distance had done us in. That first gravity-altering kiss, though, set a standard that lasts to this day. And it definitely made me want more—more boys, more freedom, and a lot more fun. I was sliding into my own version of "girl gone wild."

Eleven

Liftoff

I had just two goals during my final year at Bishop's: to secure a place in college and to find a date to the prom, now that Tom was out of the picture. College was the easy part. Even with the enticing distractions of men and hormones, I managed to stay on the honor roll, thanks to my deep ease with science and math. I couldn't quite wrap my mind around history, and I struggled a bit with physics, but I'd learned that most blocks would yield if you did your homework and put thought into problems. Out of habit I could still do that.

I knew I had the grades, and the extracurricular activities, to land a spot at a good school. My mom pushed for Harvard—she wanted nothing less than Ivy League, preferably the crème de la crème. I gathered applications for Yale and Princeton, too, but I'd already decided where I was going: Mount Holyoke in Western Massachusetts, one of the Seven Sisters. Through my church I'd met a woman, Mrs. Bodenstab, who had the life and glowing essence that I wanted: She was refined, well spoken, and a doctor, with a perfect house in La Jolla, a doctor husband, and a beautiful boy and girl. She introduced me to Mount Holyoke at her alumnae gatherings, where I saw photos of the campus and fell in love with the castlelike dorms.

We didn't have the money to visit, so everything I knew about the school was based on photographs, brochures, and the sense of refinement I got from Mrs. Bodenstab and her friends. I think I also had enough insight into my adolescent self to know I'd be better off at a school with no men than on a coed campus. Bishop's, though it had been coed for more than a few years by the time I got there, was still run by women, a distinguished and formidable group I respected and admired. I figured that was something it might have in common with Mount Holyoke and that I wouldn't suffer if I had academics as a main course with boys on the side. I applied to the school that looked like something out of a fairy tale.

I asked for an early decision and got my answer in December when my college counselor, Mr. Leander, a round, exuberant man, ran through the crowd of students on the sidewalk near the quad, waving a piece of paper. "You got in, you got in!" he yelled, lifting me off the ground. It was a good thing, too—I'd only sent in one application. I could've scrambled to get in somewhere else, but essentially my Plan B was the same as Plan A: Get into Holyoke.

Mom was disappointed I hadn't given myself a shot at Harvard, but I was happy to have freed myself for an entire spring of senioritis. I had finished the most advanced science and math courses I could take, had my quota of credits, and now only needed to lock down the prom date to make my year complete.

I didn't really have to look far. Roger, the orderly who'd taken me under his wing when I started candy striping in the emergency room, had begun paying attention to me in a more grown-up way. Thanks to the confidence I'd gained with Tom, I could return his flirtatious gestures and jokes, and I made a big deal of turning seventeen in the spring. It sounded a lot older than sixteen. Roger was twenty-four, almost twenty-five, and I knew I was young for him, but I didn't care. I could see him for what he was: six foot three and handsome, with an angular face, green eyes, and shaggy brown hair. He was smart, he surfed, and he loved medicine. Not to mention the way he'd mentored me through my time in the ER. Why would I not go out with him?

My mom could've listed her objections from then until this moment—and she would've been right. Roger drove me to Tijuana and into the rough-and-tumble of the bar scene and took me to parties with his friends. I'd been a straitlaced girl, the level-headed one who could always see the consequences. But with Roger I wanted to linger in the moment and not look ahead. It was a big shift for me, the one who never got in trouble.

On one particularly memorable night, Roger and I drove to a party in La Jolla, where his friends had hired a good Latino band to play. I'd never drunk alcohol before, so when someone handed me a sweet cocktail, I gulped it down and asked for another and another. The band was sounding so good to me that I walked up to the lead singer and tried to join in. The band humored me for a while, but when I planted myself at a microphone and wouldn't leave, they began to lose patience. Then I demanded "Louie, Louie" and belted out a slush of words that were even less comprehensible than the real ones.

"Hey, you better go get her," someone told Roger.

"Holy shit, she's plastered," he said, sounding surprised. I think he'd thought I was just pretending to be drunk.

He'd been drinking, too, and that made his friends' next suggestion—driving around with the windows down till I sobered up—sound reasonable.

"Let's go for a ride, Lisa," he said, putting his arm around me and leading me to his van.

"Yay!" I said, leaning on him heavily and pushing his arm up to my shoulders when it dangled to my chest. And then I threw up on his shoes.

"Tell me you didn't just do that," Roger said, as his friends laughed and backed away.

It was a long ride back to La Costa.

"I knew I was stupid to get involved with you," he said. "I am such an idiot." He banged the steering wheel with the heel of his hand and stepped on the gas. I scooted to the far edge of the seat and tried to disappear. For a while he seemed to be yelling at himself, but I got it that he was also yelling at me, and when he arrived at "and this is just too crazy. I can't date a girl like you," I realized that those drinks had pretty much left our relationship on the deck.

"Does this mean you're breaking up with me?" I asked.

"Hell, yes."

"You can't!" I sobbed. "You have to take me to the prom."

"The prom? Let's just not talk right now, okay? I'm getting a headache just thinking about it."

Mom was asleep when I got home, so at least I didn't have to explain my ruined eye makeup or my unsteady walk. I'd never been drunk before, and it wasn't working out for me. I couldn't see the point of it. The bed spun as I tried to sleep. For the next few days I called Roger over and over, pleading with him to just keep going out with me till the prom was over. Then we could break up if he was still mad at me.

"Look, you won't even sleep with me," he said. "I've been patient, but this isn't going to work if you won't."

I held him off and kept repeating my party line: Just stick around till after the prom, and then everything will be negotiable. It seemed to buy me some time. After my next shift in the ER, we went out again, and he said he'd missed me. He even joked about my drunken disaster at the party. On prom night he showed up in a tux.

We raised a lot of eyebrows at that prom. A seventeen-year-old girl didn't look quite right on the arm of a twenty-five-year-old man, even if he was a cool, smart surfer on his way to med school. "We were concerned about Lisa's escort," the headmistress of my school said when she called Mom the Monday after. "How old was he? We don't think that's appropriate or good for her."

Mom used her nicest bureaucratic demeanor to say it was none of the school's damn business, but when she got off the phone, she sounded just like everyone else. "He's a lot older than you are," she said, "and he's going to have you doing things you wouldn't normally do with friends your age. That's trouble."

"Don't worry, Mom. I won't get in trouble."

"You will throw everything we've worked for out the window if you get pregnant," she said. "You know what these older guys expect."

My friend Christina had an older boyfriend, too, and she didn't make it to the prom with him. She was pregnant and about to leave school. I did know what older guys expected, but it wasn't what I wanted, and if nothing else, Mom had raised one headstrong daughter. I wasn't about to take my eye off the goal I'd had since I was a little girl—not for a guy. Certainly not for sex. Roger and I dated until I left town, but we drew the line at anything that might produce offspring. A relationship with a seventeen-year old wouldn't look good at USC, where Roger had gotten into med school. And I had no intention of winding up like Christina.

I squeezed in one more bit of eyebrow-raising activity before I graduated. The spring was a long countdown to college for the senior class, with a "hundred-day" party to set the mood when we were three months from graduation. That was supposed to be followed by senior ditch day, a free day off for our class. But a couple of kids had gone hunting after the big party, and one had been killed when a gun accidentally discharged. Our class was small and close, and the whole school was in shock and mourning for weeks.

Eventually, though, someone looked up and said, "Hey, we didn't get our ditch day!" A guerrilla plan evolved to claim it by going to a Padres baseball game. We figured that if enough of us went, we couldn't possibly get in trouble. But apparently, we didn't achieve critical mass. When I got back to campus, I found out I'd been suspended.

What might've been a disaster earlier in the year was a misdemeanor at this point, though, and all was quickly forgiven. I threw my cap into the air and settled into going out with Roger and selling contact lenses at a mall to save as much as I could for college. The funny thing about growing up with Mom and her peculiar relationship to money was that when I applied to Mount Holyoke, it never occurred to me that people don't go to the colleges they want to because they can't afford it. I took out a student loan and figured I'd face the reality of repaying it sometime down the line. Growing up without money, you know you'll sign your future away and spend the rest of your life figuring out how to pay it back. But "the rest of your life" is far, far away.

I knew there was no chance that Mom would step in to help me out. The signs I recognized were showing up again. We'd moved a couple of times, edging farther and farther from San Diego, and she was beginning to spend more time on the phone with Grandma talking about Christopher's needs. He was having trouble keeping up with the kids in his preschool, and his teachers thought he'd need special schooling. Mom's demons were still there for her to battle, too, usually in the form of some person or other who was "out to get her" at work. Grandma was sending checks again. Close as Mom and I were, I could sense that we'd crested and were headed for some kind of descent.

TWELVE

Meltdown

I didn't own a pair of socks when I landed in Massachusetts, and even when the snow fell in drifts, I preferred to let it slide into my boots and freeze my bare skin rather than confine my toes. I was cold all the time, but going sockless was part of my California-party-girl persona, which I honed, to predictable effect, during my first year at Mount Holyoke.

I was initially paired up with a black roommate, but we rubbed each other the wrong way from the beginning, in part because I wasn't ready to be "segregated" with one of the only other black women at this new school. So I made friends with a small group of girls from Minnesota in my dorm and some California girls from another dorm. The California girls took me to my first campus party, and this time there was no Roger to keep an eye on me and see me home. I danced all night with my sunglasses on, my soon-to-be trademark move.

When I finally got home, I could've slept all day, but I had a job interview to get to, with a family in South Hadley, our college town, that was looking for a babysitter. It wasn't easy, but I pulled myself together and got there. I was relieved to land the job but not so relieved when tensions intensified with my roommate, who wasn't happy when I kept going to parties with the Minnesota girls. I was doing the kind of things a lot of normal sixteen-year-olds would do. But my "normal" was different from other people's, and

I was finding that out the hard way as I was exploring life away from my mom for the first time. One of my Minnesota friends, Amy, a fellow premed student, stepped in and worked out a roommate swap so we could share a room—no big deal.

She had no idea.

True to her Midwestern roots, Amy was Miss L. L. Bean, with curly blonde hair to her shoulders, frosty pink lipstick, and cute pink or green wool sweaters paired with turtlenecks, some printed with tiny hearts. She was neat and preppy, the "you betcha!" opposite of jaded. Our room was set up with a narrow bed, dresser, and desk on each side, mirror images that quickly devolved to the Martha Stewart version of heaven and hell. Amy's half was flawlessly decorated in her preferred pink and green, and she had a place for everything, from her perfectly folded sweaters to the neat piles of books on her desk. I was more of a "leave it where it lands and rifle through the heap" organizer. By the end of the first week, my desk and bed were buried under clothes and Coke cans, and the surfaces never reemerged. I had never learned to fold clothing or organize anything domestic. I taped a surfing poster sloppily to the wall and called the decorating done.

Academics weren't much of a problem my first term. My calculus class used the same text I'd had during my senior year of high school, my French was good, and I didn't have any problem keeping up with the reading and writing for English. Biology was a surprise—much harder and faster moving than what I was used to, so I was paired up with a study partner, a brilliant blind girl who wound up tutoring me. That class kept me interested, but for the most part I was coasting. School rolled on in the background while I turned my attention to boys, parties, and campus life.

Mount Holyoke was a women's college, but that didn't mean there weren't men; it just meant that the men were imported. A bus made the rounds of the five neighboring colleges in a loop that took about twenty minutes to cover, so it was easy to visit back and forth, and students from even farther away came in for parties. Amy and her Minnesota friends and I went to a series of mixers, and at one of them Amy met a Dartmouth guy named Bud who caught her fancy. Bud, athletic, tall, and a star of the baseball team, introduced me to his roommate, and as a matter of convenience, the roommate and I paired up. The four of us went to a couple of parties together, but I found the roommate somewhat odd, and when it came to kissing, he didn't come close to my dizzying Tom Darby standard. There wasn't a hint of chemistry between us.

Bud seemed to be having the same reaction to Amy. He took me aside at one of the parties and stood very close.

"Lisa, what's Amy been saying about me?" he asked.

I laughed. "You're great, you're cool, and she really likes you."

"Shit," he said.

"Come on, Bud. What do you want her to say? That she worships you and wants to have your baby?"

He didn't crack a smile. "I just . . ." He paused and leaned toward me to whisper in my ear. "I just don't feel that way about her, you know?"

His breath warmed my whole body, and if I'd turned my head slightly, I could've kissed him. I wanted to, but I didn't right then. A smart girl wouldn't have done it at all—but I wasn't terribly smart that year. Bud pursued me with calls and notes, and I wound up getting involved with him just long enough to betray Amy and then—instant karma—realize he was going out with a girl at his own school.

I ruined my relationship with Amy, and many other girls in the dorm stopped speaking to me as well, much the same way the people in our church so long ago punished Mom for getting involved with the preacher who sought her out. This male-female thing wasn't going to be easy. I hated the way Bud had fooled me, and I hated what I'd done.

I ostracized myself when I realized nothing I could say would make things right again. I tried to spend as little time as I could in the dorm and stayed in the library until it closed, slipping into the room when Amy was in bed. I even quit eating in my dorm dining room during the week, though I worked there waitressing and washing dishes. Not using my meal plan meant that I could only afford one meal a day during the week: a tuna melt, French fries, and a vanilla shake from a snack bar. On weekends I ate alone in the dorm, but I retreated if I saw the girls from Minnesota. I wanted nothing more than to disappear.

I was doing things Mom's way that year, not thinking about the consequences of my actions until I was drowning in them. It didn't work for me. I lost my babysitting job because I called my mom from my clients' home. I don't know how they felt when they found out about the long-distance charges—money was the least of it. While I chatted with Mom, the little girl I was supposed to be tending kept coming over and asking if I'd take her to the basement. I was so starved for a dose of Mom that I kept the girl waiting until her father, who I'd assumed was gone, came bounding up the basement stairs. He fired me on the spot, and I knew I deserved it. It was another wakeup call. I'd so hoped to stop being "the responsible girl" I'd been all my young life, but I was beginning to see how she'd protected me. She was the one who knew, deeply and truly, that I couldn't live with the turmoil of being like my mom. And both that responsible part of myself and the wayward rest of me were relieved when harmful acts had consequences.

I was desperate to get home by the time Thanksgiving rolled around. I'd been so homesick I called Mom almost every day until the first bill came and the phone in my room had to go. After that I'd waited near the hall phone for her calls, but my "exile" made it hard for me to do even that. I booked the cheapest flight I could find, a string of short hops with long waits in between. The trip took twenty hours.

Things in La Costa were much as I'd left them. Mom and Christopher were still living in the smallish apartment we'd had, and Mom, as far as I could tell, was doing all right. The phone worked, the car was in the garage, and Christopher was turning into a chattering little whirl of energy. But Mom seemed down, even though I knew she was thrilled to see me, and we spent the holiday chasing our four-year-old, watching old movies on TV, and eating takeout. I was a little embarrassed about the fuss she made over me in front of Christopher, but I soaked it up all the same.

I was eager to see Roger, whom I still considered to be my boyfriend even when Bud was in the picture, but when we met at his apartment near USC, our visit was strained. Now that we weren't working together, we seemed to have nothing to talk about, and he stiffened when I tried to put my arms around him. I went back to Mount Holyoke with that typical freshman feeling of belonging exactly nowhere.

A note from the resident advisor of my floor was waiting for me when I returned. I was being summoned to a meeting of the dorm administrators, resident advisers—and Amy. I think the adults knew I couldn't go through another semester of isolating myself and trying not to live in my dorm. It was bad for my mental health, and there was no relief for Amy, who still had to live with my avalanche of stuff. Amy was friends with everyone on our floor, and they'd all taken her side, or at least I imagined that they had. I would've. So in this divorce she was getting the room—I'd have to move out at the end of the term.

Hard on the heels of getting kicked out of my dorm, I got a note from Roger saying he was breaking up with me. And when I went home for Christmas, there was more change in the wind. Mom picked me up and took me to a hotel in Carlsbad instead of to the apartment. She'd gotten us a gorgeous suite right on the beach, and we were practically the only guests, but it didn't make sense, even extravagant Mom sense, to spend that kind of money for that kind of place at Christmas. Something was up, but she wouldn't tell me what.

"You are such a worrier, Leese," she said as I warmed myself by the abandoned pool in the thin, hot rays of the winter sun. "Just relax."

Some freshmen might've taken the opportunity of a new semester to regroup, and I set out to do just that. I'd take a deep breath, give up men and partying for a while, and dig into my classes. I went back to school for the optional three-week winter term and signed up for ballet and a women's theater class. But I was no match for the dark and cold of the Massachusetts winter, and I wound up repeatedly calling in sick for my theater class because I dreaded the freezing walk across campus. That ended when I went to the gym to work out and spotted someone whose shape looked vaguely familiar to me with my contacts out. When the shape came closer, it turned out to be my theater teacher—who gave me one last chance to show up. I took it, but the lesson I learned—don't get caught!—wasn't one that would help me with my fresh start.

My first semester troubles, paradoxically, had gotten me into one of the dorms I'd fantasized about. Unlike my first room, which had been in a disappointingly modern building, my new one was in North Mandelle, which, just as in the brochures I'd seen, looked like a castle. Perhaps because of my sockless surfer look, I stuck out on campus, and at North Mandelle my reputation had preceded me—I was the girl who'd gotten kicked out of her first dorm.

My new roommate, a premed junior, didn't care, nor did the girls I met on my floor when everyone came back to campus for the spring term. I took up with a transfer student named Marianne from the Netherlands and three other girls, who became the close-knit tribe I'd been craving since I arrived. We clicked immediately. Marianne was a fun-loving, artsy girl with a generous bent, and when her family sent her a jar of Nutella, the chocolate-hazelnut spread she'd grown up eating, our little group devoured it. We named ourselves Nutella, because we fancied ourselves exotic, like this European treat. And also a little nuts.

The Nutella girls were my poison. We'd straggle to class and meet for dinner to plan our evenings—parties, concerts, frat functions, trips to 7-Eleven in our nightgowns. We began to come in so late so regularly that we stopped sleeping in our own rooms and took over the living room of the dorm, where we kept alarm clocks to rouse us for the last of breakfast. With events on five campuses to choose from, we could go out every night. I'd never had freedom like this before, and I was determined to make the most of it.

Toward the end of the term, the Nutella girls decided to go to see Cheap Trick at a huge outdoor concert at UMass in Amherst. I wasn't a fan—I knew just one song—but I was happy to tag along. We found a spot not far from the stage where we could see perfectly until a linebacker-size guy muscled into the space in front of us. I tapped one of his massive biceps.

"I'm just a little girl, and you're blocking my view," I said sweetly. "Do you think you could move over?"

He stared at me. "That's funny, little girl," he said, turning back to his friends. He could easily have moved over half a foot, but he planted himself and didn't budge.

I couldn't believe I couldn't charm him into sliding over. "Come on," I said. "I just need a window."

He ignored me. "Don't be a jerk," I said. "We were here first." Nothing.

And that's when I began to yell and call him names. Before I knew it, a beefy security guard was walking toward us. "Miss," he said, "come with me."

"See, little girl," the linebacker guy gloated. "Now you're really in trouble."

My friends called after me, saying, "You don't have to go with him!" but I stayed behind the security man. We got closer and closer to the stage, and when we crossed a barrier at the front edge of the crowd, the security man said, "Robin Zander saw you out there, and he wants to meet you." He pointed to some stairs leading to a wing of the stage behind a stack of giant amps.

Not being a Cheap Trick fan, I didn't know that Zander was the band's lead singer, but when I got to the top of the stairs, it wasn't hard to figure out that the guy in tight jeans and red-framed sunglasses who'd walked toward me from a cluster of musicians and roadies was in the band.

"You like my music?" he said. I nodded. He had long blond hair and a lot of swagger. He was around Roger's age, maybe a bit older.

"Oh, yeah," I said. He was cute.

"You want to stand on stage during the concert?"

"Yeah, sure," I said with a big smile.

He walked back to his guitar and I stood just offstage, waving to my friends, who had been certain the security guy was taking me to detention for the fracas in the crowd. The linebacker looked stunned.

I danced through the whole concert, visible to everyone, and when it was over, Zander asked if I wanted to go to an afterparty at the Howard Johnson's up the road, where the band was staying.

"I'm with some friends," I said.

"Girls?"

I nodded.

"Bring 'em," he said. "Call this number when you get there."

Without thinking too much about what we might be getting into, we drove to the motel and went up to the room, a plain, slightly trashed little suite, with a couch, a desk, and pair of queen beds. I made a beeline for Zander. Marianne hung back at the door, and when I went to get her, she was edging out. "Look how old these guys are," she said. "Let's go."

"Oh, come on," I said. "We can't just leave now."

Robin rested his hand on the bare skin of my back.

"You're gorgeous," he said, wasting no time. "I love the way you dance, and I'd like to get to know you. Why don't you come with us?"

I wasn't practiced enough to recognize a cheap pickup line or, as the band might've put it, a cheap trick. I said something about being a student, with finals coming up, but he shrugged that off.

"Listen, I'll send a limo for you, and you can meet up with us. You work it out." His hand had moved up my back to my neck, and he was pulling me closer when Marianne showed up at my side.

"Hey, Lisa, we have to get back," she said. To this day I thank her for that.

Robin winked at me. "You call and tell me where to send the car tomorrow, okay?"

A limo did pull up outside the next day, but I phoned Zander and said I had to finish up my classes. He paused, then asked me where

I'd be spending my break. "We're headed for LA," he said. "Let me give you the number where we'll be. You can meet us there."

I was innocent enough to believe him. I arranged to take my finals early so I could go to the LA show—the only initiative I'd taken in my classes all term. I'd managed to ace my first semester without studying, and I assumed I could do it again. I could always fake my way through English and French, but my calculus class had moved into territory I hadn't covered in high school, so I'd devised a plan for working around that. There were a couple of cute high school boys taking our class for advanced placement credit, and I'd befriended one of them, inviting him over to the dorm to study. I could tell he was flattered, and it was easy to get him to not just help me with my homework but to do it for me. I'd drop into class occasionally, at first, but by the time of the final, I had no idea where we were in the book—which was especially unfortunate because it was an open-book test. Long afterward, I replayed the nightmare feeling I had when I walked out of the exam. I knew I deserved to fail. It only made things worse that I'd used that sweet, hopeful boy.

I got the first C of my life in that class and Bs in the rest. Suddenly I was a 4.0 girl with a GPA that started with a 2—it was almost unfathomable. Deep down I knew what GPA had to stand for next term: Get Productive Again. And I knew what the C was about as well: Consequences.

When I got to San Diego, I tried calling Robin's LA number, but the woman who was always on the other end kept telling me that he wasn't available and I'd have to leave a message. On the fifth or sixth call, I finally asked her: "Are you sure he's getting my messages?"

"I'm telling you, he knows you're calling," she said. I just wasn't getting the hint.

Thirteen

Cheap Tricks

I think I clung to the fantasy of hanging out with a rock band because reality closer to home had turned grim again. Mom had put all our belongings in storage and scaled back to a small place in downtown San Diego, not far from her office. Something must've happened or she wouldn't have moved again, but she wouldn't tell me what, and I didn't press her. I knew how much energy it took for her to keep the juggling going for Christopher and me and how her mind never stopped trying to solve the Rubic's Cube of her finances. When she let her guard down, she might talk about how she wished she could just start over with a clean slate. But times were tense again, and she wasn't letting me in.

She'd used her work contacts to line up three jobs for me, enough to keep my share of the tuition paid for another semester. I cobbled together as much financial aid as I could, but each term it was a stretch to cover everything, just as it had always been. The summer jobs were mind-numbing, but I was glad to have them.

Monday through Friday I got up early and drove Mom to work, dropped Christopher off at day care, and went to my job at a contact lens company, where I worked as a file clerk and tried to stay sane as I demonstrated my incredible mastery of the alphabet. At five I'd go pick up Mom and Christopher, change my clothes and run to my second job, as a waitress at SeaWorld, a purgatory of fish sandwiches and kids with sticky fingers. On the weekend I'd dress

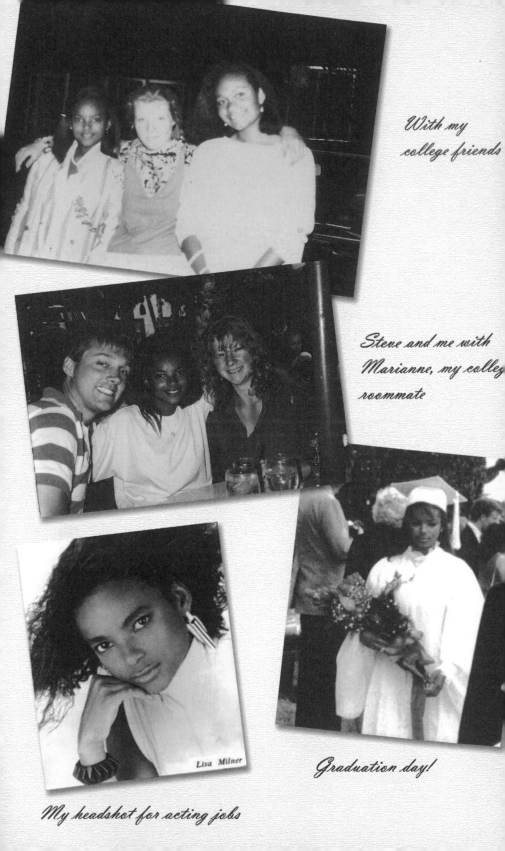

*With my
college friends*

*Steve and me with
Marianne, my colleg
roommate*

Lisa Milner

Graduation day!

My headshot for acting jobs

up for my shift as a coffee girl at the Hotel del Coronado, a classic Victorian beach hotel with an upscale clientele. I had Sundays off, but I was too tired to do much besides sleep.

With no time or energy for partying, I thought a lot about the upcoming year. Late in the spring my love life had completely crumbled—I was still smarting from being dumped by Roger and Bud. Much like my Mom, I tended to see what I wanted to see and assume that I could make it happen, and I was slow to realize that you can't just will men into staying with you.

But I'd lucked onto a guy who seemed to genuinely like me, no stretch of the imagination necessary. I met Steve Masterson at a party my roommate dragged me to, to meet some guys from Amherst. He was an all-American type with sandy brown hair and gray-blue eyes that kept catching mine after we were introduced. I walked away to dance, but he followed me and stuck by my side. We left the party together that night and dated, first casually, then almost exclusively, until I left.

Steve was a philosophy major with an eye on law school. He was a couple of years older and a lot less wild. I'd promised him that I'd say goodbye before I went home for the summer, but when I took off early, we'd missed each other. He came by my room with flowers, but I was already gone. Still, I held out hope that I'd hear from him because I'd given him my address and he'd promised to write. But as the weeks passed, no letters arrived. I fantasized about how I'd get serious about school and let him be a good influence on me in the fall, but I had a feeling I was in Robin Zander territory again and I'd missed my chance.

With or without Steve, something had to change—I despised myself for the C in calculus and the men who were suddenly so easy to attract and so hard to manage afterward. At the end of the term, when the Nutella girls put in bids to live in a suite we could all share sophomore year, I'd opted out, and asked for a room in another building with a serious girl I knew. I was even ready to buy a few pairs of socks.

I took it as a good sign when Mom told me at the end of the summer that there was some mail waiting for me at her post office box. She'd conveniently forgotten to mention that, when she left La Costa, she'd rented a box near our old house. I figured that meant she hadn't been sure at the time where she was going or how long she'd be there. The PO box was so far away from the new apartment that she rarely went to check it—any bills collecting there were just one less thing to worry about. But she'd finally gone, and the box was crammed with letters from Steve.

I was so glad to see them I didn't bother to get angry about how Mom had let them be abandoned. I arranged the envelopes in chronological order and read them in one sitting. The first notes were chatty and affectionate, but as the weeks wore on, the tone became more and more upset, asking why I hadn't responded and speculating that I'd let my silence do the talking for me and I was breaking up with him. I wrote him immediately to say I was sorry and that I'd explain what happened when I got there. I hoped the "Love, Lisa" would be a tip-off to where he stood.

Before I went back to school, I asked Mom if we could stop at her storage unit so I could pick up a few things. She hadn't made a move all summer to reclaim any of our belongings, and I had a feeling that I should take anything precious with me, just in case. Home for me had always been wherever Mom was, but my gut told me it was time to shift my base to college and think about my future. Maybe I'd actually try to become a doctor.

FOURTEEN

Spiraling Up, Spiraling Down

Steve was solid, sexy, and right within reach. And I had a stack of letters to prove that he'd not only thought of me during the summer but was anguished when I didn't reply. So at the ripe old age of eighteen and a half, having dated only a handful of guys, I decided he was the one for the long run.

I wanted someone who knew me well enough to be a safe harbor, a buffer between me and the chaos I knew was just below any calm surface I could create. If that makes our chemistry sound underwhelming, it wasn't. Steve took that role so willingly, and so naturally, that I marveled. He was an easy choice for me, and we were a good match. He felt like home to me. I wrote out our names and combined them. Lisa Milner Masterson. It sounded like who I'd always been.

"You still have that dream of going to med school, right?" Steve asked me one day early in the fall.

"If I didn't blow it last semester," I replied.

"That wasn't you, it was that Nutella phase," he said. That made me laugh. "You're smart, you'll claw your way back. I'll help—I'll study with you."

I signed up for a full load of premed courses. I'd liked my biology class, and now I was adding chemistry, more math, and more French and English. Steve didn't seem to have the workload I did, or maybe philosophy just looked easier because he didn't have formulas and equations to master. But he was happy to sit and read Kierkegaard as I pored over homework.

Actually going to my classes put a lot more structure in my days than I'd had freshman year. I took jobs for money as well, grading science papers and answering the door and phone at the bell desk of my dorm. And after dinner I generally headed for Steve's room, a single in the Theta Delta frat house at UMass in Amherst, a twenty-minute bus ride away. I was there studying as often as I was in my own dorm, and I got to know all his frat brothers. I kept in touch with Marianne, my Dutch friend, but now when we went out, it was to grab something to eat or take a walk across the campus, where the maples were flaming red and we were surrounded by a postcard-perfect New England fall.

Steve and I went to his family's home in Pearl River, New York, for Thanksgiving. Steve's dad was a professor at Rockland Community College, and his mom kept the household running. They were a perfect *Leave it to Beaver* nuclear family, with Steve and his older sister Martha. The house was neat and quiet, with china dishes, gravy boats, huge trees in the yard, and bedrooms that were shrines to the childhoods that had passed there. If my being black had caused any turbulence before I arrived, no traces remained when we arrived for the late afternoon meal. They'd gone all out for my visit: I found out later that Steve had pushed his dad to put in a new bathroom upstairs for me.

That term I found my footing, my old intensity, and my grades shot up. I finished with a GPA back in the 3s and an invitation from my biology professor to work with him on a research project that I'd be able to turn into a thesis and probably publish. I began to think I might be looking at a career in biochemistry if I didn't wind up in medicine.

Mom was the only cloud in my turnaround year. I'd been worried about her since I'd gone back to school, and I knew she was in trouble when I got home for Christmas. She looked fine, and she seemed like her old self, but she had moved Christopher to yet another apartment, a dark, tiny place in Coronado. It had been six months since she'd put most of our things in storage, and she still hadn't taken any of them out. For the first time there was no bedroom for me, so I slept on the couch and counted the days until I could go back to my dorm room. Christopher still had learning difficulties, and Mom had him in special programs that must've cost a fortune.

When I went home for the summer, I packed a suitcase but left the rest of my things in storage at the dorm. Mom was living in the same building, but from the looks of things, all hell had broken loose when I left. I felt as though I'd let her down. The place had filled up with clutter—bags of papers, old clothes, and even trash were piled up, and Christopher's toys were strewn everywhere. Christopher seemed to come in and out of the jumble and not notice, but it was shocking to me. We'd never been neat, but Mom saw to it that our places had at least a touch of order. That was gone. Mom was probably depressed. She slept more than I remembered, closing the door to her room and disappearing, with my little brother still sitting in front of the TV. She was a mother who needed a child who could raise himself. I think she'd expected Christopher to be like me, and that was something he just couldn't do.

I had my same roster of jobs—filing at the contact lens place, waitressing and pouring coffee at the hotel—and as exhausting as that was, it was more stressful to come home at night. Mom didn't try to explain herself, and when I asked about her job she wouldn't go into detail. "You know how it's always been, Leese," she told me. "A black woman's got to fight for everything she has." As usual, everyone was gunning for her. At least that's what she told me.

My uncle Don, who spent a lot of time with her when he was posted to San Diego during that time, says he thinks things were finally beginning to catch up with her. "Your mom always did whatever she could, whatever she needed to do," he told me a long time after. "She wasn't beyond embellishing—and she did. It was one of those classic cases. They didn't verify her résumé, and she had to operate above her level of competence. She could exist on cunning and skill, but it took a lot out of her." I could feel how stretched she was and how close to ripping the scrim on which she'd kept her professional image afloat. She still carried home her briefcase, but she hardly ever opened it. Her weight had crept up, and every ounce of her sagged.

A couple of weeks before I had to go back to Mount Holyoke, Steve was coming to pick me up for a trip up the West Coast, the first time he'd been to my part of the country—and the first time he'd be meeting my family. This place was certain to scare him off. I hauled bags and bags to the trash and scrubbed as much as I could, but the kitchen was so dim and dingy that I couldn't bear the thought of bringing anyone, especially Steve, into it. Not after seeing where he'd grown up.

If I'd known anything about paint, I might've just given the walls a fresh coat, but the thought didn't occur to me. What caught my eye were some festive rolls of contact paper I passed at the supermarket, white with yellow flowers. I brought home an armload and peeled and pressed until I'd covered the whole space, even remembering to cut out a rectangle for the light switch. There were bubbles and tiny wrinkles here and there, but overall I was pretty pleased with my first big home-improvement project. Then Steve walked in.

"You know that's contact paper, like for drawers," he said politely as he looked around. I hadn't known at all. We'd never lined a drawer with anything, ever.

"It's cheerful though, right?" I said. By the end of our road trip, my wallpapering attempt had become a joke between us, but I still can't think about contact paper without wincing.

"There's one thing you should know about Lisa," Mom told him, stating the obvious. "With her you're getting a companion. She doesn't cook, and she doesn't do housework."

"Yes, ma'am," Steve said with no further comment. I loved him for that. He loved Mom, too. They were both quick with a quip and fiercely protective of me.

I found lots of reasons not to go home in my junior year. Steve had started law school at George Washington University in Washington, D.C., and I had immersed myself in my thesis research project, which needed constant tending. My biology professor and I were studying a neurotransmitter called norepinephrine, which not only passes impulses from one nerve cell to the next but also comes into play when the body is under stress, helping produce the "fight or flight" response. We were mapping the pathway it traveled in the brains of mice to get a better understanding of how it functioned. It seemed like a serendipitous topic, the mechanics of stress.

Our "mapmaking" was a two-year process that took many hours a week. We wanted to attach a molecule of nickel to the norepinephrine so that when we injected mice with it, then studied their brains with a scanner, the metal would light up, showing us the path the chemical had taken.

I hadn't spent much time in the lab, but now I was there all the time, sharing a chemical bench and a small cage of rats with my mentor. His reasons for helping me may not have been entirely based on my enthusiasm for his classes—he had a reputation for trying to get close to his female students. But I was in love with Steve, and it was easy for me to keep things cool and professional.

Our first task was to figure out how to combine the neurotransmitter with the nickel and get a substance that was both stable and nontoxic to mice. If that sounds complicated, it was. We came up with a number of stable combinations, but a lot of our rats didn't survive them, and for one discouraging period, I watched my cages getting emptier by the day. Finally, though, we had our tracer.

Mastering the biochemistry and producing our non-lethal neurotransmitter took us a year, and by the end, I'd fallen in love with research. I began looking into an internship at the National Institutes of Health in Bethesda, Maryland, where I might be able to get a sense of what a career in the lab would look like. I could've done that in Boston or any number of research facilities around the country, but the NIH was close to D.C., and Steve and I wanted to be together.

I spent the summer mixing chemicals, and though I managed to get to Washington for occasional weekends with Steve, I was almost happy he was away so I could immerse myself in my last year on campus. I was working on a French thesis as well as the one in biochemistry. My advisers said no one had ever done two and warned that, if I did, one wouldn't be accepted, but I told myself that if mine were good enough, they'd make an exception. So under the guidance of my French professor, a charming man from Senegal, I began working on a project that traced the development of civil rights movements in several colonized African countries through literature written in French.

In the lab we'd reached step two of our research: injecting our mice with the nickel tracer we'd developed. We wanted to watch them experience the effect of the neurotransmitter and then study their brains. For that we'd need to slice the brains open, freeze them with chemicals, and put the frozen tissue through an electron scanner.

I landed an internship at the NIH to learn the freezing technique, and after Christmas at Steve's, I spent my school's winter miniterm working among professional scientists. It was as dazzling to me as my first encounters in the emergency room in San Diego, and I could imagine myself on the front lines of a field that would produce cures, not just administer them. Steve and his roommate were living in a small, cheap row house near Union Station. The neighborhood was moderately dicey, but it felt safe when Steve was on my arm. All of us were swamped with studying, but Steve and I soaked each other up.

I wrapped up my research in the spring and presented it to the college's science board, showing slides of the chemical formulas we'd used and scans of the mouse brains. After they gave the thesis high honors, my adviser admitted he hadn't been sure I'd ever be able to get to the point of collecting data on my first time out. I couldn't persuade anyone to accept my work in French as a thesis—though I did get a great grade in the class.

The glow of it all didn't last. All that traveling to Washington, time in the lab and accumulation of books for my research had cost money I didn't have. Late in my last semester as I tried to check out of the bookstore, I was bluntly informed that my student credit account was empty. I demanded to see the manager, but there was no budging him. No money, no books. If I wanted them, I'd have to pay up my tuition for the term. I was almost surprised that the argument "but I was too busy studying to work!" didn't have an effect. This was college. We were *supposed* to be studying.

There was no way Mom could help me out, and I couldn't borrow from Steve—he'd know I could never pay him back. So I did the only thing I could think of: I went to the headmistress of the school and told her how desperate I was. I wept as I told her I hadn't been eating because I couldn't afford to and how even though I was going to graduate with honors, my mom was too strapped to come to my graduation. "It's killing her," I told her, sobbing. By the time I left her office, the headmistress had wiped out my tuition bill for the last term and offered to fly Mom to the ceremony. But I walked away thinking, "What just happened? That's not me—that's Mom!"

I feel queasy now about how easy it was to embellish the story, just the way Mom would've, with drama and tears. Now I understood from the inside how she'd kept us afloat all those years. It was my saving grace that I'm a notoriously bad liar—my face is an open book—and that my relief at having the burden lifted was marbled with guilt. I didn't have a lot of "Mom moves" left in me. I decided to choose another way.

Fifteen

Proposal

Mice trump flies. People trump mice. And a guy with a diamond ring trumps most other people. I knew that much by the end of my first year out of college. High on the reception I'd gotten for my mouse-brain work, I wanted to try on full-time research as a possible career, so I went back to the National Institutes of Health. They were glad to have me, but for many reasons it wasn't a great fit.

For one thing: the flies. I was assigned to a scientist who was working with the DNA of *Drosophila*—the fruit fly. To get the DNA you need a lot of flies—and not just the random crowd you get by leaving overripe bananas on a counter. My boss's research depended on flies hatched from eggs we spread over agars (those gels you see at the bottom of Petri dishes) made of peanut butter. I was responsible for making sure our eggs and young flies were well fed and happy in their heated glass enclosure, a clear column where they could meander through the air in what I hoped would be growing numbers. The flies aren't fast, so it wasn't much of a problem to keep them contained when I opened and closed the drawer that slid into their space to feed them. But I could always feel them circling.

The other part of my job involved looking at the DNA we extracted by subjecting a slurry of flies and chemicals to an electric field. That process causes the DNA to form visible lines on the gel that results, and those lines were the heart of our work.

We were crammed into a small office, the flies and gels and I, and I spent hours serving peanut butter snacks to the insects, peering at the lines on the gels, and occasionally talking to my boss about what we were finding. About three-quarters of the genes for human diseases have a match in fruit flies, so *Drosophila* DNA has been used in research on Alzheimer's, Parkinson's, and a host of other conditions—I knew this was important work. But I could've wept with boredom. Lines and flies, lines and flies. I started retreating to my desk, tucked into a nook behind our work area, and calling my mom for long chats. She was a government worker, and now so was I, and I assumed that the government phone plan must surely feature unlimited calling.

I'd also walk down the long hall connecting the science wing of the NIH building with the hospital on the other side. I felt almost physically pulled toward the familiar rhythms of need as medical workers and patients moved past. I decided to take the MCATs, the medical college admission tests, and apply to med school.

On my short list was Hahnemann University in Philadelphia, a school known for its holistic approach to medicine. Steve was in his second year of law school, and the firm where he'd interned during the summer had snapped him up—unless he got a better offer, he'd be working there, in downtown Philly, when he graduated in another year. I assumed we'd be together, though we'd had a tough time in D.C. I hadn't planned to share his apartment when I went back to the NIH, but I had no luck finding affordable housing in a neighborhood that didn't scare me. I pleaded with Steve to let me squeeze into his room again, and we rationalized that it would be fine. Both of us were out of the house all day and into the night, especially with Steve setting up camp in the library to keep up with his studies. But we got on each other's nerves in such close quarters, and I reverted to a bad old pattern. Whenever he mentioned the name of a female student, or introduced me to a woman he knew, I'd feel pangs of jealousy and then berate him for being untrue to me. Stressed and insecure, I was a piece of work.

A wild card popped out of the deck as I was bemoaning my decision to turn my life over to the care and feeding of small insects. I was window-shopping in Georgetown when a well-dressed woman stopped me, introduced herself, and asked if I would be interested in modeling. "You have an exotic look," she told me. "Where are you from?"

I could tell she was trying to place my ethnicity, but I didn't feel like helping. "California," I said.

"Have you thought about modeling?" she asked. It had to be obvious that I'm only five two and not really cut out for the fashion world, but she persisted anyhow.

"I don't know," I said. "I'm on track to go to medical school, and I have a job. I don't really have time."

"Well, think about it," she said, handing me her card.

I stuck it in my pocket and straightened up as I walked down the street. I'd always been supremely confident about the "smart" side of myself, but the "woman" side, the one that would turn heads if she were self-possessed enough to believe she could, still looked in the mirror and half expected to see a chubby little girl with ugly glasses. If nothing else, this model scout's card was something I could pull out when I felt fat and ugly to remind me that things had changed. But I really didn't have time to pursue the fantasy.

Steve didn't see it that way.

"What, are you nuts? You have to go check it out," he said when I told him about the chance meeting. He looked the company up in the phone book. "See, they're legit," he said. "You get a couple of jobs and maybe you could pay for med school. Go talk to them."

I set up a meeting at the modeling agency and went to hear the pitch. The Georgetown office was staffed by attractive women and lined with large photos of models. The woman I'd met on the street introduced me to the agency head, and they explained that height wasn't really an issue for TV commercials, which is the work they'd try to get me. Med school was a nonissue, they added. If I got just one national commercial, my tuition worries would be over. They sent me to have head shots taken at a warehouse studio where I got to toss my head in the wind of a fan and smile. Apparently, my tossing passed the test. They signed me to a contract and connected me with a New York agent, and before I knew it I was in a trade-paper ad promoting the agency's "up and coming" talent.

I didn't believe anything would come of it until the agency started sending me on calls for commercials—in New York, a long, long train ride from D.C. One of my first auditions was for a Sprite commercial, a cattle call where everyone in the room was going to be reciting the same three lines. I had no idea what to do, and at my agency all they could tell me was "Just be bubbly!" So when the clients called me in, I was as effervescent as I could be, feeling the whole time as though someone had tossed me into the deep end and yelled, "Don't forget to smile" as I was going down.

I was always disappointed when I didn't get the job. After all, it wasn't rocket science, or even a thesis. What people told me was that I didn't look as though I felt comfortable in my own skin, and it was true. Eventually, I'd wind up there, but it was something I'd have to earn.

I juggled my auditions and the lab until my boss called me in and let me know he thought I was getting distracted. He also wanted to talk to me about something else—those phone calls to my mother had been sky high, and though they weren't going to dock my pay, I couldn't make any more long-distance calls. I was stunned. I'd been positive that calling her office from mine would be as cheap as using

Dixie cups connected with string, and I was mortified to see how much I'd "spent"—especially since I couldn't offer to reimburse them. Independent as I felt then, I'd shown in bold red ink how much I still needed my connection with my mother.

It was a tremendous relief when I got my letter of acceptance from Hahnemann. I didn't have the dedication to flies or the lab-bound rigors of research to stay at NIH. I needed to be with people, and I'd veered away from my original path only because my thesis work had been so successful at every step. But my thesis didn't have to be my life. I'd learned firsthand how much basic science and research supports the work of doctors—and now I could leave most of that discovery process to someone else.

Steve landed an internship in LA for the summer, and my mom used her connections to get me a job at Neiman Marcus selling women's clothing. We traveled down to see her on the Fourth of July weekend, but almost as soon as we got there, Steve started talking about taking a trip to Catalina Island. Mom was living in the same building in Coronado, now in a brighter upstairs apartment. Things were still cluttered, and the tumult of living with a little boy was still evident, but this wasn't the disaster area we'd found the last time I was home, and I couldn't understand why Steve was so eager to leave.

"I know Mom's place isn't what you're used to," I snapped, "but can't we just try to enjoy being here?"

"Honey," he said, "when was the last time you went to Catalina? It's beautiful. We'll just make a day of it and come back."

I rolled my eyes. "We just got here, Steve."

"You two just go," Mom chimed in. "I don't think I told you that I'm taking Chris to play ball with some kids from church, and I don't think you need to do that. We'll see you for fireworks."

I was being railroaded, and I alternately ranted and pouted for the entire ninety-minute ferry ride to Catalina. I was still complaining as Steve put me in a rented golf cart and drove us up the road from the dock. He seemed to be looking for something, and we circled aimlessly until we reached a grassy spot overlooking the glittering blue of Avalon Bay. Steve jumped out to spread a blanket, and for the first time I noticed the beautiful woven picnic basket he'd been lugging. He laid out a lunch of wine, cheeses, and fruit, and I grudgingly climbed out of the cart and sat down. He put his arm around me. The grumbling in my brain tried to start up again, but it was impossible not to relax into the setting. A cool breeze tempered the heat.

Below us church bells began to ring. Steve hopped up and reached into the basket, pulling out what looked like a sock. He unwrapped a small velvety box, dropped to one knee, and with bells still tolling said, "Lisa, you'd make me the luckiest man in the world if you'd be my wife." A diamond glittered from the dark case. "So that's what this was all about!" I said, finally smiling. "I mean, yes. Yes, of course!"

It wasn't a complete surprise—we'd gone as far as diamond shopping a couple of months before—but it was the last thing I expected that day.

It was the sweetest of coincidences that when we got back to the dock to wait for the ferry, we ran into my old prom date, Roger. My new ring flashed as I reached to give him a hug. "Roger," I said, savoring the words, "this is my fiancé, Steve."

Steve and Lisa the engaged couple were a lot like Steve and Lisa the settled-into-dating couple, except that now our place was filling up with bridal books and magazines, which I devoured in every spare minute, making notes and dog-earing pages. Work was far less absorbing by comparison. I found the ladies who circled through the racks at Neiman's about as interesting as *Drosophila*, and it saved my sanity that a diversion appeared. My New York agency connected me with an LA agent, and I began getting calls to audition for movies, which I found extremely odd, considering that I had never claimed to be an actress. But I was happy to try, on the off chance I'd land a job that might help pay for med school. I would've considered being shot out of a cannon if there was a chance it would cover the cost of a semester or two.

It might be a comment on the state of the movie business that I got callbacks twice that summer. Steve tried to coach me for a role as a "common woman" in a period piece. But he was no help at all when it came to the beer ad the agency found for me. Glancing around at the Pamela Anderson look-alikes, I could only think I was truly in the wrong place. I think my life was trying to hint that there might be a way to meld medicine and some kind of media, but it was early for that—I needed to handle the "become a doctor" part first.

Sixteen

Anatomy, and a Wedding

Med school was a shock to the system. My entire academic career had been built on classes that were scarcely larger than ten or twelve people, but at Hahnemann, most of my first-year classes were lectures delivered to the entire freshman class in a huge auditorium, with only occasional small-group classes and discussions. I was a tiny cog in an elaborate machine where every other cog was one of the best and the brightest.

The first two years were an onslaught of information, and the sheer amount of work in the first year was overpowering. I'd had difficult classes before, but with so much to absorb in so little time, I felt as though there was no way to keep up. Classes started first thing in the morning and continued until five or six in the evening—at which point I'd study frantically to try to retain what I'd seen through the windows of the speeding train.

With Steve back in Washington to wrap up his last year of law school, I moved into a dorm a block from campus. It could've been anywhere, considering that I scarcely looked up from my books and the stacks of notes I got daily from a note-taking service. I woke every morning to a tape of Robin Williams yelling "Good morning, Vietnam!" which seemed to sum up the state of siege. For the first time I tried drinking coffee, but the caffeine gave me heart palpitations, so sheer will had to serve as my NoDoz. A sweet guy named Paul Schnur lived down the hall, and he'd knock on my door after dinner, when I'd showered and put on a flannel nightgown, to quiz me and go over notes. He and my friend Racine, a sharp black woman with beautiful green eyes, kept me company for the marathon of memorization.

I'd met Racine when we sat next to each other in a lecture, and I figured her for a ditz. But when the results of our first exam came back, her score was much higher than mine. I couldn't believe she was so smart. She had a different system from mine of going through material, highlighting this, underlining that, and I scrambled to work out my own technique. Lots of people were in study groups, but they seemed like a waste of time to me. I had to struggle through a few more exams before I realized I needed to learn new ways to learn.

My roommate was in our program, too, but we weren't a perfect match. She was a little spoiled, and when Steve came up to visit, she'd parade around in a shirt and underwear. I tried to keep my distance.

I came home one evening to find she'd taken a phone message for me: "Your agent says you have an interview for *The Cosby Show,*" she said. She was incredulous. "You have an agent? And you've got an audition for Cosby?"

When I'd told the agency I was moving to Philadelphia for med school, they'd offered to put me up in a house with some of their other "talent." I'd been firm about having less than no time to audition, but I'd been seen once by the Cosby people when I lived in Washington, and this was the equivalent of a callback. Philadelphia was just an hour and a half from New York by train (as opposed to the four-and-a-half-hour trip from Washington), so I gambled on one last audition that might pay for my schooling.

When I arrived at the call, I noticed that the other people in the room were a lot younger than I was, so I went to change into a more casual shirt, and when I got back, someone handed me a script. With no coaching about the character, and precious little time to study the lines, I went in to read for the part—Theo's girl-friend. When I didn't get it, I got back to the business of studying—and felt lucky to have gotten that distraction out of the way early.

I hated the grind of memorizing, but I was enthralled by gross anatomy, that odd and sobering encounter with the body. The pre-served skin and bones and muscles of the cadaver in front of us were foreign and familiar, and here, working in small teams, we first felt the sharpness of our tools and the intricate layering of the body that revealed itself to us bone by bone, system by system, organ by organ. Our cadavers were wrapped in towels and stored in coffinlike metal cases, with sides that dropped down to reveal a person we'd never known but would come to know very well. I remember the whiskers on the face of our body, an older man. I'd pause sometimes and wonder if his soul might still be nearby. Is this how we all end up, I'd ask myself, empty and becoming emptier by the day?

Most of the time, though, I was absorbed in looking at the body from such an intimate vantage point. One mark of doing such close work was that we were greasy all the time—the body's fat had liquefied and clung to us, along with the powerful smell of formaldehyde. It permeated our clothes, hair, and skin, and it was nearly impossible to remove. Sometimes Steve would come home late and head for me, only to veer away. "You didn't already take a shower, did you?" he'd say. "You might want to put on some scented lotion." That embalmer's smell and the scent of curry, which wafted through my dorm from the room of an Indian stu-dent who lived down the hall, linger in my memory as the strange perfume of that year.

It wasn't easy to squeeze wedding planning into my schedule, but I did my best. Steve and I had invitations printed at a big Philadelphia department store, and his sister Martha came down from New York one weekend to help me find a dress. My other huge decision, where to have the wedding, was an easy one to make. It would be at either St. Mary's Chapel on the Bishop's campus or St. James, where I'd been an acolyte. A quick consultation with my Princess Diana fantasy for the big day settled it: We'd go with the larger St. James, where I'd lighted so many wedding candles over the years.

I went home to San Diego after my finals in May to pull everything together. I had just a matter of weeks and minimal help from Steve, who was starting his job in Philadelphia.

Without a father to foot the bill, I called on every resource I had to finance my vision: I ran through the meager sum in my savings and checking accounts, took out new credit cards and charged them to the max, and kept Mom in reserve in case I ran into trouble. I ordered flowers from Adelade's, the best florist in town, and had my bouquet fashioned after the one carried by Grace Kelly, my wedding muse. I wanted the church filled with white flowers—tuberoses and lilies—that were as sweetly scented as they were beautiful. For the reception I decided on the Westgate Hotel in downtown San Diego. The hotel's aptly named Versailles ballroom, with its cream and gold interior and glittering trio of Baccarat crystal chandeliers, would be our setting. We'd have a hundred guests and a bridal party of six groomsmen, to accommodate Steve's friends and fraternity brothers, and six bridesmaids. My social circle was smaller than his, and I worried about finding six people to fill the pink dresses I'd chosen, but a combination of high school and college friends came through.

I tasted samples from the hotel's menu, thinking less about cost than how much I liked the food. Steve agreed to handle the engraved menus and place cards, and since he was paying for them, he turned an economical eye to the frills. "Hey, those little bows cost $1.50 each. We're not getting them," he told me. When the stationer called to double-check the order, though, I was the one who answered the phone, and bows were back. What was $1.50? I didn't tell my husband-to-be about the Versailles until the invitations were in the mail.

As I tasted and ordered my way through the planning, brandishing my credit cards with abandon, Steve got to be a nervous wreck. But qualms about the cost didn't hit me until I got a call from the hotel reminding me that my fifty percent deposit was, after all, only half the fee. The rest, $7,000, was due in full five days before the wedding. And I didn't have it. I hadn't wanted to involve Mom in any of my creative financing, but with the wedding party beginning to trickle into town and the plans firmly locked down, I caved. When I told her about my predicament, I could see cogs beginning to spin behind her eyes. "We'll figure this out, Leese," she said.

I applied for more credit cards, which I instantly maxed out, and Mom called Emmett, my ex-stepfather, to see if he could help with the rest. It would just be a loan, she assured him, something for old time's sake. I wanted to say, "I'm not sure you'll ever get this back," but instead, I just said thanks. We were just three days from the wedding when we finally had all the money.

There was last-minute drama, of course. On the day of the ceremony, the only black hairdresser in the area, miles from La Jolla, kept me waiting so long I was almost late for the ceremony. I had to dress in the bride's room of the church, and after all that, it still took some deft touches from my mom's comb to make my hair look the way I'd envisioned it. She rushed me out of the room, my

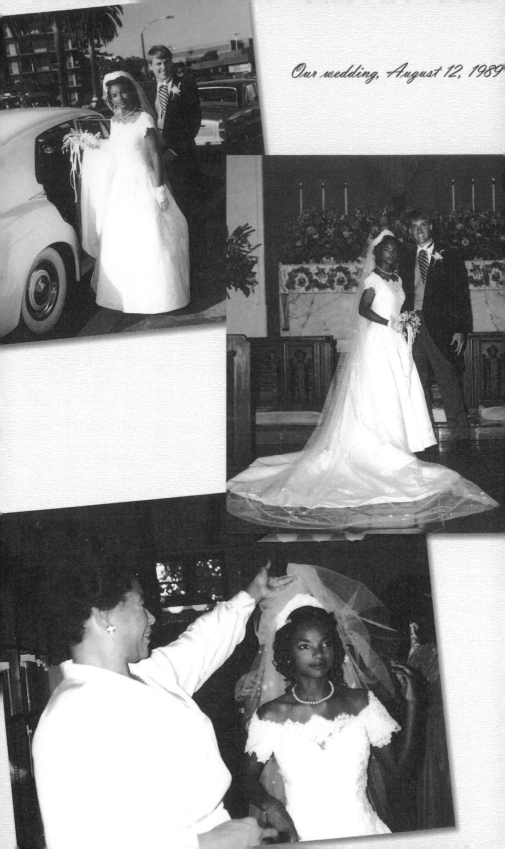

Our wedding, August 12, 1989

uncle Almer walked me down the aisle, and miraculously, Steve and I got to "I do."

We rode to the reception in a Bentley that one of Mom's friends had arranged for us, and when I walked into the Versailles ballroom, it had been transformed in just the way I'd imagined, with magical arrangements of flowers and candles. We feasted and danced, and on the first night of our marriage, we collapsed into bed, wanting nothing more than rest.

Steve's gift to us was the honeymoon, a ten-day trip to Moorea and Bora-Bora in Tahiti. He'd arranged for us to be met by a hydrofoil that would let us skip the two-hour bus ride to our hotel, and as we stepped from the craft, people asked who we were. We felt like Mr. and Mrs. Bond. It was a fantasy, just as the wedding had been.

I know extravagance like that seems crazy, but looking back on it now, I feel a lot of tenderness for that young woman who felt so driven to have a fairy-tale wedding she couldn't afford. For that one beautiful day, all the pictures she'd been cutting out of magazines to create a collage of what might be were no longer "trash." They were reality. I'd met a man who loved me, and our grand wedding was proof that we'd make a life whose wonders weren't just glued to a piece of cardboard.

Soon enough we'd begin the hard part: putting in the years of work that would make Steve a successful lawyer and transform me into a doctor. But for that one day, and that brief honeymoon, we could taste what it would be like when we arrived. I was building a family, and there would be bedrock under our feet. I could look around me and see it. The scared, doubting part of me could relax and believe.

Seventeen

Crashing

Things fall apart. That's the theme of the second year of medical school, when the focus shifts from how the body works to how it breaks down. My whole life that year seemed to pivot around breakdown—and bits of hard-won healing.

Steve and I flew straight from the South Pacific to Philadelphia, taking just a week to set up housekeeping in our new home, a small townhouse a couple of blocks from the campus. With Steve's old bed and sofa, a new dining room table and a random assortment of wedding gifts, we did all the decorating we had time for. We stuck a cot and a bedside table in one of the three tiny bedrooms and called it a guest room, left one room empty, and arranged our meager belongings in the rest of the place. Immersed in my world of disease, drugs, and microbiology, along with Steve's black hole of billable hours, we barely glanced at our surroundings. Home was a place to study, sleep, and eat ramen or takeout, the extent of my kitchen repertoire.

Smaller classes and the study skills I'd picked up my first year made it easier to pack facts into my brain, but marriage didn't have the desired effect on my psyche. Instead of feeling secure about Steve's love for me—the guy had jumped through an inordinate number of hoops to get to "I do," after all—I struggled with jealousy whenever he mentioned another woman. That may have had something to do with the thoughts I was trying to squash as I looked around at my classmates. Some of them were very smart men, passionate about medicine—and extremely cute. Guys would see my diamond and jokingly complain about how someone had gotten to me before they could. I didn't play out any attractions, but I couldn't honestly say I hadn't fantasized about it. And if I was feeling that way, Steve probably was, too. Sometimes that was all I could see. It's funny how hard it can be to take in what other people tell you, even when it's "I love you." I had to learn to hear it and believe.

We were arguing when we got into the car one day that October, yelling at each other as Steve ran a stop sign a block from our house, and a Mack truck slammed into my side. I felt as though someone had picked me up and hurled me into a brick wall. The pain was blinding. When the roar stopped I turned to Steve and said, "We've been hit." I was having trouble breathing.

The door and frame of the car were crushed around me, and it seemed to take hours for the police and fire teams to pull me out of the wreck. Steve wasn't injured, but he was terrified for me. The emergency room doctors worried that one of my lungs had collapsed and cut off my clothes to get at the damage. The lungs were fine, but I had two broken ribs. Neighbors who'd seen the crash were astonished to see me walking around just a few days later—I was some kind of miracle. I took two weeks off from school, nursing my bruises and the deep ache in my right side as I tried to study. Life had just screamed "Stop!"

We were so gleeful about being alive that everything seemed easier. I memorized slides of diseased tissue and immersed myself in the workings of viruses and bacteria and the drugs that fight them. Steve slid into the rhythm of office politics and casework. Jealousy seemed trivial for a long while as we restarted our life together, seeing this second chance for what it was: a blessing.

I thought Mom was checking on me again when she called in early December. I'd tried to downplay the seriousness of the accident, but as soon as she heard "Mack truck" every protective impulse ignited, and she touched base with me even more than usual. That day, though, she wanted to talk about herself.

"Leese," she said, "I went for a checkup today."

"That's great, Mom," I said, "I know how you hate doctors."

"Leese, they found something . . . on my mammogram," she continued. "It's not good."

Mom had always been sturdy, and she was only fifty-one. My mind pulled up those facts as if they could save her.

"What does the doctor say?" I asked.

"I could get a lumpectomy or they could take . . . my whole breast," she said slowly. "I want you to come hear what he has to say."

"Let's not even talk about anything drastic. We'll go see him together, and I'll help you decide."

I flew out on my holiday break and sat with her as the doctor spelled out the pros and cons of removing the breast versus removing just the malignancy and following up with radiation. My grandmother was adamant when we called her: "Get that disease out of you," she said. "Let them have the breast. Let 'em have the other one, too. You can't fool around with cancer."

The thought of Mom losing a part of herself scared me—I thought "disfigured," the same reaction I'd had as a kid when the bad relaxer job had made her hair fall out. The feeling was visceral, completely bypassing my med-student brain. But I tried to be neutral: "It's a big decision, and it's up to you, Mom," I told her. "The doctor isn't pushing one or the other."

I was relieved when she chose the lumpectomy, and I stayed with her through her first radiation treatment. She was as calm and optimistic as I've ever seen her. We'd been through trouble before, and we'd get through this. I was sure of it, and she seemed to be, too.

I was so wound up when I got home that Steve and I decided to get away for a weekend in Atlantic City. "Honey, how about if we have a baby," I said. The logic of the moment said, "You've been together for years, you're married. What's next? A family." We were a modern two-career couple, but somehow—maybe it was all those old movies I watched as a kid—I seemed to be imprinted with the life vision of a '50s wife. We didn't analyze it or think too long about why the baby idea was surfacing right then. Did the accident or Mom's condition have something to do with this? It didn't come up. We decided it was time, and our odds were stellar: We succeeded on our first try.

I kept my pregnancy to myself as long as I could, but I had to tell Racine when we were assigned to draw blood from each other in one of the increasing number of modules designed to prepare us for dealing with patients. "You go first," I said. I had no problems sticking a needle in someone, and candy striping had accustomed me to the sight of blood. But when it came time to hold out my arm for her, I refused.

"I'm nervous about this," I said as she began to wrap a rubber cord around my arm.

"You think I liked having you aim for a vein?" she said.

"No, really, I don't think I can do this," I told her.

She gave me a look.

We sat there at an impasse until I said, "Okay, I didn't want to tell anyone, but here's what's going on. I'm preg. . ."

"You're what!"

"Shhh. I'm pregnant, and I'm not sure what they're testing this blood for. I don't want this to come out on a blood test. I'll tell them in my own way."

"You haven't told the school?" Her eyes were wide.

"What could they do about it anyway? I'll handle it."

I rolled down my sleeve and Racine found another blood donor. It was true that I was worried about a possible pregnancy test revealing my status too early, but the greater truth was that I'm squeamish about my own pain. I didn't want an amateur aiming a needle at my arm.

We learned to do pelvic exams thanks to the generosity of women who volunteered to let us make our first clumsy attempts. With great skill they gave precise feedback as groups of four or five students probed for the cervix or ovaries. They were so in tune with their bodies that they could let us know exactly what we were touching and what we'd missed.

I admired their matter-of-fact grace because right then I had so little. You never surrender as a control freak, and so I struggled, feeling trapped in a body taken over by aliens. The more I learned, the more out-of-control things seemed. I could hardly sit through our unit on pregnancy and delivery. Where the job of an ob-gyn giving prenatal care is to reassure the mom-to-be and give her confidence about how things will go right, my classes focused on diagnosing problems and cataloging what can go wrong. The message: Pregnancy is riddled with risks. But even without breaches, breaks, tears, or toxemia, I realized I was in trouble. Watching a video of a normal delivery, I felt stricken. "How in the heck is this kid going to come out without damage?" I thought, resting my hands on my rising belly. "This is really gonna hurt." I'd known that rationally, of course, but presented with the howling and bloody face of birth, I wanted to rewind the clock and reconsider. Other people seemed moved by the sight of new life coming into the world, but all I could think was, "How did I get myself into this horrible mess?"

I was lucky to have few symptoms to deal with at first—mild nausea but no real morning sickness—but my experience was more "grimace and bear it" than "glowing with motherhood." As the baby grew my body began retaining water and sent me looking for restrooms at the most inopportune times. I'd never been so uncomfortable. And as time went on, things only got worse. It was as though I got every odd condition I'd studied. Splotchy brown spots appeared on my face: the mask of pregnancy. My salivary glands amped up their production, and I felt as though I were drooling. I got rashes and then bad acne. My voice even began to deepen (I learned after I delivered that I'd had an ovarian cyst that caused my body to amp up its testosterone production). I was a textbook case for any number of irritating conditions. But pregnancy is time-limited, and there's a sweet reward at the end. I clung to that thought as I lumbered through.

We started to look for hospitals, and when we didn't like the one close to Hahnemann, we decided to move to Bryn Mawr, on the Main Line, where we found not only a good facility but also an apartment that would give us access to a lawn and lots of room for a child. Steve and I would have to take the train into the city, but it seemed like a worthwhile trade-off.

We decided on a name then, too. We'd call the baby Daniel, after Steve's father. We were lucky it was a boy—for some reason we'd never been able to settle on a name for a girl.

Spontaneous as our decision to have a baby had been, we'd been realistic about my schedule. Years three and four of med school put you on clinical rotations in the hospital wards and operating rooms, observing and learning basic procedures in a series of specialties. The schedule was designed to be flexible: We could take our two months of summer vacation anytime during the last two years of med school. I would do the first rotation, use my vacation time to have the baby, then jump into the program again. At least that was the plan until I walked into the maternity ward for my first rotation, obstetrics and gynecology. A nurse took one look at my swollen body and said, "I want to take your blood pressure." It was frighteningly high. There would be no rotation for me, at least until I saw my doctor.

The news wasn't good: I had preeclampsia (the name given to the high blood pressure that arises during pregnancy), and my doctor ordered me to stay off my feet. Regular hypertension drugs could put the baby at risk, so rest was the first-line treatment. My blood pressure and liver functions would have to be closely monitored, and there would be regular ultrasounds to check on the baby.

As I fought off worry—about Mom, about the baby—I slowly began to embrace the idea that I could take the year off instead of running to catch up with my class. I'd have time to be a wife and mother, and maybe, for a change, I'd just rest. I'd been driven from the time I was old enough to go to school, always trying to achieve and reach out of myself for something just beyond my grasp. I was so tired. Maybe it was time to just be. Steve was thrilled. I think he had a '50s fantasy himself. He'd be the man going off to work, and at least for a while, I'd be the stay-at-home mom.

A week before my due date, I began feeling contractions. I called my doctor and headed for the hospital. It was a false alarm—I wasn't in labor—but my blood pressure was off the charts. "Today's the day," the doctor told me. "I don't want to take any chances. We're just going to keep you here and induce you." He began a drip of medication to bring the pressure down but soon decided that both the baby and I were in so much danger I'd need an emergency C-section. If I'd been terrified before, the operation put me in shock. With my arms positioned straight out from my torso, I felt as if I were on a cross. And then someone came at my abdomen with a knife.

That's the point of view you don't have as a doctor. I've done hundreds of C-sections by now, and the memory of my own is never far from me. Awake, and in the midst of surgery before my epidural had fully taken effect, I was in intense pain. We obstetricians generally tell women that after the epidural they'll feel some tugging and pulling but nothing more. I make a point of trying to keep that promise.

"Just let me see his face and then knock me out," I told the doctor as I struggled against the pain. "I need to see his face."

I woke in the recovery room, throbbing and angry. I looked at the baby and thought, "What the hell! I went through all that for *this* thing?" I went back to sleep, and I stayed in that enveloping darkness until the next day.

The nurses tried again. Did I want to see the baby? I shocked myself by spitting out a "No, I don't." But the staff instinctively brought me a photo of him and got me into a wheelchair to take me to him. Daniel wasn't in the nursery. He'd been rushed to the neonatal intensive care unit after breathing in some meconium during the delivery. Meconium is a tarlike substance that lines the baby's intestinal tract, and when it's inhaled, it can irritate the lining of the lungs and cause breathing problems. He was doing fine, but he'd be in the NICU for another four days.

I looked at the tiny, beautiful being in the incubator and began to feel a surge of love.

Eighteen

Luck

"If I didn't know you were my child, I wouldn't recognize you on the street," Mom said when she saw me in my hospital room.

"I gained so much weight I look like Jabba the Hut," I moaned. We both laughed. Mom always cut to the chase, and it was a refreshing relief.

She'd hopped on a plane as soon as Steve called to tell her about the emergency C-section, and though she couldn't be there for the delivery as we'd planned, she was sitting beside me when I woke after the surgery.

She stayed for a week, cooking and cleaning, and when she left my mother-in-law arrived, bringing me food and preparing a couple of weeks' worth of meals that we could heat in the microwave. Their help had never been more welcome. I felt as though I'd been hit by another car—or maybe a train—and for days I could hardly get out of bed.

Daniel seemed healthy when we finally brought him home, but before we left, the doctors gave us one more thing to worry about: The small birthmark on his left cheek, an irregular, rosy patch, was probably just superficial and likely to fade as he got older. But there was a chance it was a symptom of neurological problems. It hadn't occurred to us that there might be something seriously wrong with our baby, and now we were full of worst-case scenarios.

Things intensified when we took Daniel in for his first pediatric checkup. "I'm sending you to a pediatric neurologist," the doctor said. It was a jolt. We grabbed the first appointment we could get and tried to hold ourselves together as we waited for the expert's opinion. But the neurologist was smiling as he walked toward us in the waiting room. "It's just a birthmark," he said. Finally, we could get on with being an ordinary family.

I still had some emotional distance to travel before I could bridge the gap between my fear and loathing of pregnancy and the closeness I'd hoped motherhood would bring. I didn't resent the baby, but I didn't feel the connection everyone said I should have. Eventually, though, it came. Several weeks after Daniel was born, I cinched him into a baby carrier on my chest and went to the market to pick up a few things. All of a sudden I had the feeling of being watched. I looked around and didn't see anyone, but when I glanced down, there was Daniel, his dark eyes smiling up at me. His look went all the way through my body, and right then I fell in love with my baby.

From that moment on I had the bond I still share with my son today, and I'll always treasure the gift he gave me with his penetrating gaze. It was pure love.

I couldn't get enough of doing for him. I—Miss "I don't do cooking"—was happily slinging pots in the kitchen for the first time, making baby food from scratch. I even rejected Pampers in favor of cloth diapers and smelly diaper pails. (That lasted until Steve picked Daniel up one morning for a good-bye kiss and the baby peed all over his suit. Superabsorbent padding never seemed like a better idea.) I'd wheel Daniel to the park to see the ducks, and like moms through the ages, I became a regular of a department-store photographer who'd pose my dressed-up boy with bright toys and give me packets of portraits to send out to everyone I knew. Daniel and I were at the train station every

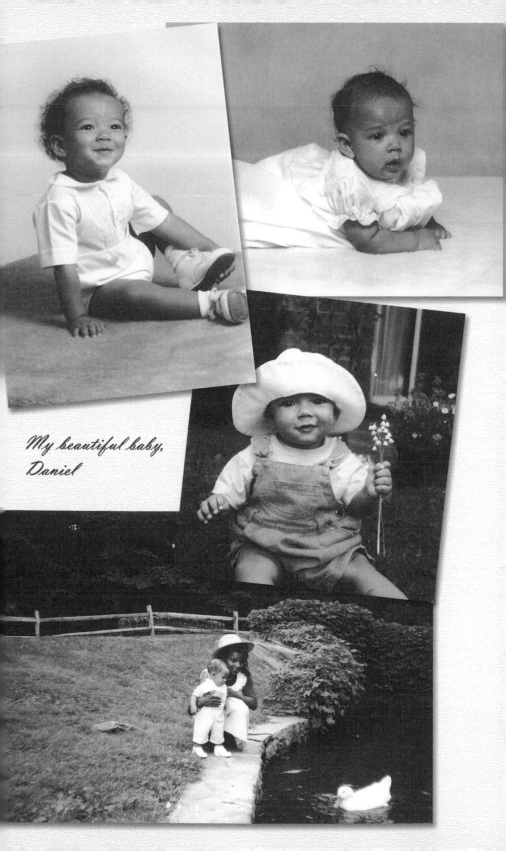

My beautiful baby,
Daniel

evening to greet Steve. I didn't want my men to miss a chance to be together.

I was surprised by how much I enjoyed my days. I knew my time off was finite, so I reveled in it. The only real task I set myself was to lose the weight I'd gained and get back in shape. My brain snoozed in baby time, and for the first time in years I got some rest.

Mom's cancer came back in the spring; this time she'd get a mastectomy. "I knew they should've done that the first time around," my grandmother said, taking no pleasure in being right. I took Daniel to San Diego so we could be with her for the operation and the first of her treatments. It was a difficult time—Mom started becoming sensitive to the radiation after just a few rounds, and her tissues swelled. I grieved to see her lose the breast and to see her so uncomfortable. But she was stoic and as cheerful as she could manage. She was good at the placid surface, but it was hard to tell what was going on underneath. Joanne, a friend of hers who had two small boys, had been taking care of Christopher; no one talked about what was going on at work. It was hard to go back to Philadelphia.

"Honey, I've been thinking about applying to USC to finish out med school," I told Steve when I got home. "I know it won't be easy, but with Mom like this, it's what I really want."

He practically snorted. "You want to do this now? Are you serious? Well, (A) you're probably not going to get in. It's the middle of the year, and you'd have to be at the top of your class for them to take you. And (B) remember my job? You know I didn't make any great connections in LA the first time, and it's not going to be easy to do it from scratch. I won't even have an internship. Why can't you to fly back and see your mom instead of making us move out there?"

"I just wanted to let you know I was thinking about SC—it means a lot to me," I said.

"Not gonna happen," he replied, turning on the TV and staring at the screen as he flipped through the channels. "I can't even think about it right now."

It was case closed, as far as he was concerned, and I let it rest. But I was worried about Mom, not just her health but everything else. She'd been struggling to juggle the finances even without the medical bills and the time off for her treatments. She'd listed Christopher as Samoan to get him a good spot in one school program for help with his learning problems, and who knew what bills she was neglecting so she could pay for his golf lessons. She wanted him to thrive at something, and golf—never a cheap sport—was what he seemed to love.

I couldn't let go of the idea of going back to California. Getting an MD from USC had always been a dream, especially after Roger got in, but I hadn't even considered it because of Steve's job. Now that I had time to think, I wondered why I'd given it up so easily. I began to obsess. It didn't help that after spending months with Daniel, I was starting to go buggy. I loved being a mom, but motherhood wasn't the only thing that defined me. I needed to be a doctor, not just for myself but for Mom and all we'd done to get me to the brink. I called USC and asked them to send me the application materials. Steve was probably right—it wouldn't be that easy to get in. But you can't win if you don't play. I typed up my CV, gathered up my transcripts, and sent everything off. I didn't bother to tell Steve.

Cocky as I'd been, the arrival of the acceptance letter threw me. "What do I do now?" I asked Mom in a frantic phone call.

"Well, you're stuck now, aren't you?" she said.

"Oh, God, Mom."

"You need to figure out what you want to do," she counseled, none too helpfully.

"Mom, you know what that is," I said.

"Then you'll have to work it out with him."

"Work it out with him" was not exactly what I did. When Steve got home I held up the letter. "I know you were skeptical about this, but I got in," I said. Steve looked at me as if I were speaking Greek and his mind was struggling to catch up.

"I'm thrilled about this," I said, heart pounding, "and I need to be with Mom. I know it's hard, but she needs me so much now, honey. I have to go."

"Wow," he said. "Wow."

The baby and I flew out to stay with Mom in late August. Steve regrouped and began putting out feelers at LA firms, saying he'd come when he could.

Mom's hair had fallen out and was growing back thinly under her wig, but otherwise she seemed fine, more tired than she'd been when I saw her last but on her feet, recovering. A few days into our stay, I put Daniel in a car seat and drove up to LA to look for apartments. I worked through the ads I'd circled in the paper, concentrating on Eastside neighborhoods near the campus. I stopped to make a call at a convenience store, and we were parked outside when I heard screaming and someone came running out the door. The place was being robbed.

I'd just gotten back in the car, and I'd missed being in the store by just a minute or two. I scrunched down below the steering wheel and hoped that no one would see me. Daniel, thank God, was napping and quiet.

The criminals blew past us, but being that close left me shaken, even after the police arrived. I called Steve and told him I was afraid to leave. That whole side of town seemed like the Wild West to me now.

He wracked his brain for someone who could help us and called his old friend Marc from law school. Marc dropped everything to drive over to be sure we were all right and took us to lunch so I could calm down.

Steve hadn't been in touch with Marc for months, but nothing cements a friendship like realizing who's on your short list when your family's in trouble. Marc has been one of our closest friends ever since, a connection cemented when he told Steve about an opening in his firm and offered to put in a good word. The grinding job search Steve had feared never materialized—he landed the position.

Luck is a funny thing. I think my marriage was probably saved by a guy with a gun at a 7-Eleven.

Nineteen

County

I don't think I've ever felt more antlike and overwhelmed than when I first walked into County General Hospital, the hulking white Art Deco building where I did my clinical rotations. The hospital, built in the 1930s, had some eight hundred beds spread over twenty floors and acres of wings, all connected by long, teeming hallways and interminably slow elevators. With hundreds of thousands of patients seeking treatment every year, it was one of the busiest public hospitals in the Western United States, and its emergency room was one of the busiest in the world. The care in some specialties was state of the art, and the waits were notorious. The poor and uninsured, many of them migrants from Mexico seeking care, crowded County. The hospital had traffic from Hollywood as well. Marilyn Monroe was born there. Dr. Kildare, the '60s TV doc, saw patients there. The soap opera *General Hospital* opened with a shot of its exterior. And thousands of aspiring doctors like me learned the art and craft of medicine by practicing there.

Clinical rotations are an apprenticeship, a chance to see how the information you've been amassing—biochemistry and anatomy and the mechanics of injury and disease—comes together on a living canvas. To learn the mechanical skills involved in translating knowledge to treatment, you see them, try them, then perfect them by repetition. One patient, during my first rotation, offered me an unforgettable anatomy lesson as my fingers reached into her body to locate her appendix before it came out. Others went home with sutures I'd put in or even babies I'd helped deliver. Many more felt the needles I navigated into their arms as I drew blood or started IVs. "Teaching hospital" means just that: Someone may well be learning to set his first bone or make her first incisions on you.

I started, oddly enough, in a general surgery rotation, fallout from dropping into the program midway through. Most med students steer clear of surgery on their first rotation—it's a scary way to get hands-on experience with patients. People actually considering surgery as a specialty also put it off, so they can master a few basics in other rotations and make a better impression on the surgeons teaching them. There's no way to get a surgical residency after med school if you didn't ace your surgery rotation. Surgery was practically everyone's last choice for the initial rotation, making it the most available slot when I arrived.

I wouldn't have taken odds on my survival. I was a newcomer, the only woman in my group, and the lowest of the low in the hierarchy. Training was done in teams during the two final years of med school and the four years of residency. The fourth-year (a.k.a. senior) resident coordinated care and directed the team, supervised—sometimes quite loosely—by the attending physician. The third-year (junior) resident delivered much of the treatment, backed up by the senior and the attending. The second-year resident was the junior's apprentice, handling increasingly difficult procedures and beginning to master the art of diagnosis. Below them, and under their direction, was the first-year resident, called an intern. Last came third- and fourth-year med students like me, who did the bidding of the interns and nurses.

The atmosphere was notoriously combative, a macho artifact of some ancient ritual that must've demanded tears, humiliation, and shame before a mere mortal could become a doctor. We'd listen in morning meetings as the residents and attending described a patient and told us what sort of surgery was planned. It was our responsibility to read up on the patient's condition and the surgery itself. For two months I saw mostly appies and chollies—appendectomies and cholecystectomies, gallbladder removals. Laparoscopic surgery is common for chollies now, but in those days the operation required a large incision that left a dramatic scar. My first job was to use retractors to hold open the skin once an incision was made so the senior or junior could isolate the gallbladder and cut it out. The residents would "pimp" us over surgery—quizzing us to teach us live anatomy. They'd point to something and say, "What's this attached to? What's its function?"

The pimping would continue as we went on rounds, with three or four students and a resident or an attending moving from patient to patient, discussing their cases. You might imagine a straightforward give and take of questions, answers, and clarifications. But pimping was a blunt instrument for separating the men from the boys, no matter what your gender. Answer a question wrong, make a bad guess or forget a detail of the case and condition, and instead of "Right, but you missed this" or "Study this next time," the senior resident might strafe you with comments like, "Masterson, why did you go into medicine? Do you think you should continue?" Or "How did you get here? Was your daddy rich?"

Everyone got the initial hazing, and once you'd experienced it you never wanted to be the person who didn't have the details at her fingertips. From then on, whether I was running late, hadn't slept, or had pressing family commitments, I studied my cases and prepared. It was too embarrassing not to.

In surgery my senior resident, a tightly wound Asian guy, was a man of sharply limited patience. If you were holding a retractor wrong, he'd pull it out of your hands or slap you away. Catch on too slowly, and you were done. He reduced some students to tears. My status as a new mom seemed to make me suspect—how could

I possibly be tough enough? But I began to learn. A couple of times I was allowed to reach in and feel for the appendix, and by the end of my rotation, I could step in after the residents made an incision and do an appendectomy if someone walked me through it.

My real mastery, though, came in my assigned specialty: scut work, the mundane tasks that have to be done well to keep the system humming. A maze of colored lines on the worn tile of the corridors led me from wards to labs to clinics and operating rooms, and I kept my eyes down to follow them as I ran until the circuit board of the massive hospital etched itself on my own. Med students like me were the ones you'd see racing to the lab, drawing blood, checking blood counts to be sure patients were stable for surgery, putting notes on patients' progress in their charts, and writing orders for IVs.

Almost three-quarters of the patients at County were Latino, and many spoke no English. Spanish was a survival skill, and I clung to my small medical Spanish phrase book. "Necesito una muestra de sangre"—I need a blood sample—was quickly imprinted on my brain.

I learned the small, vital ways of our world, like the need to check everything again and again. At County nothing got done if you didn't follow up, so the follow-up became second nature.

Our supervising intern checked our work and flagged lapses, often harshly. The first time I ordered a lab test stat, and then forgot about it, was the last time I made that mistake. But once we proved that we were reliable and willing to take on anything he threw at us, the assignments began to get interesting. The goal was to be the student who'd do anything—and more.

Hours were long. We were on call with the interns, so if an appendectomy came up during the night, we'd go in to assist, and the next day the attending physician, who had probably been sleeping soundly while the residents worked, would pimp us on the case.

One stroke of luck in the midst of this schedule was being able to see Daniel on my breaks. The campus had a day-care center for professors and bent the rules to accommodate us. Steve or I dropped the baby off in the morning, and it was generally Steve who left work early to pick him up when the place closed at five, since my days were so unpredictable. We were back to full-tilt stress.

During my second rotation, internal medicine, I learned that the mysteries of diagnosis, intriguing as they were, felt somehow incomplete without the hands-on work of surgery. But in my third rotation I landed on obstetrics and gynecology, which combined the best of both.

The two-hundred-bed Women's and Children's Hospital, down the hill from the main County building, overflowed with women in crisis and babies screaming into the world. The staff handled twelve to fourteen thousand deliveries a year and saw eighty to a hundred patients a day in the clinic. I began my ob/gyn rotation with gynecology cases that came through the emergency room and wound up in the windowless treatment space behind it, which we called The Pit. The long table at the entrance to The Pit was our command center. The third-year resident sat next to a phone, taking calls from the senior, who was prioritizing cases in the ER and sending them back to us. The third-year oversaw most of our work, and updated the senior on the status of our patients, whom we might be sending to other parts of the hospital when we'd finished.

The wall to the left of the table had two treatment rooms, each barely large enough for the three beds, separated by curtains, that were crammed into it. A similar treatment room was on the right, and farther back were a sink and a baby scale; an "infectious room," where we treated women with conditions that might be contagious; and a closet-size room with a bunk bed and a desk where we could lie down in the rare moments when the action slowed.

On most nights every treatment room was full, and caring for one patient inevitably meant invading the space of the woman in the next bed. Everything—the crying, the pain, and especially the sense of loss—was communal. Most of the women we saw came in bleeding, hemorrhaging from an early miscarriage or fibroids, and it wasn't uncommon for blood to pour out when we inserted a speculum. Sometimes packing the uterus and vagina with rolled gauze would stop the flow, at least long enough to let us get the woman to the OR so her uterus could be removed. Interns were trusted with the task of packing, and we students assisted, retracting or running for supplies and test results. Gurneys stacked up in the hallway, waiting for the next available bed.

I'd walk into rooms where there was blood on the walls, the floor, the drapes—it looked as though there had been a massacre every night, with one bloody procedure followed by the next and the next. In The Pit, all you'd hear was screaming, crying, panting, and the humming of the suction machine for the D & Cs, all vibrating under the harsh fluorescent lights.

We hovered to assist with the D & Cs, scraping and suctioning the lining of the uterus to remove tissue left after an incomplete miscarriage, and we collected the dead fetuses that women seemed to pass all night long in those rows of bloody beds. Late-term women were given medicine to induce the labor that would let them deliver vaginally, and the fetuses arrived large and well formed. Those we'd put in plastic bags to deliver to pathologists who'd determine why they'd died. The baby scales were for that procession of lost babies.

"Lo siento para su pérdida, señora," I'd say again and again. "I'm sorry for your loss."

Assisting the interns meant matching their pace—twelve hours on call, twelve hours in The Pit and a day shift in the clinic seeing patients. Bad as The Pit could be, I preferred it to the bottomless maw of the clinic, where we'd arrive to find a hundred women waiting to be seen by my team's second- and third-year residents, each of whom took an exam room. This was the world of workaday vaginal infections, hormone issues, and STDs, along with conditions like ovarian abscesses, pelvic infections, and ectopic pregnancies that kept women in the hospital.

Here, too, the senior resident and attending physician would check in and oversee the treatment, but the bulk of the care was in our team's hands. The waiting room would close at five, but we served everyone who had checked in before that. For students there wasn't a lot to do besides draw blood, run to the lab, and help take histories or do physicals. But the sheer numbers were exhausting.

By the time I was done with the gynecology half of the rotation, I was fairly certain that being an ob/gyn wasn't for me. I couldn't shake the sadness of The Pit, and I couldn't imagine being immersed in it for a lifetime.

But if The Pit felt like hell, the maternity ward was many flights closer to heaven, and obstetrics seemed designed to lift us in that direction. On my first night one of the obstetrics interns showed me the ropes during a delivery, describing the maneuvers the baby makes on its way out and imparting such indispensable basics as "the baby is slippery; stand close so you don't drop it." The next time around he positioned me between the legs of a woman in labor and stood behind me, hands on mine in those close quarters, to show me how to catch the baby myself. Here, the Spanish was "empuje"—push!—and "es niño," "It's a boy!" Life instead of death.

The elevator doors at the maternity ward opened onto a long hallway lined with pregnant women on gurneys waiting to be assessed by a nurse and the junior resident, who were perched at a desk at the far end of the hall with the second-year resident. They'd quickly determine who needed hydration, who was stable, who needed the close monitoring of the maternal ICU and who should go to a labor room. They kept tabs on all the women, tracking their progress: This one was stalling and might need a C-section; that one was experiencing complications and needed help stat; this one was ready to deliver.

The ward was shaped like a capital T, with the long stem of the main hallway branching into a perpendicular corridor lined with treatment rooms: the MICU, for patients with high blood pressure and other threatening conditions; the labor rooms; and an isolation room, which on various nights might hold a woman with a dead baby or a new mom with chicken pox. Tucked in back was an intern sleep room with two or three bunk beds, but no one was sleeping.

For me, experiencing pregnancy from the outside held all the fascination that was missing when I went through it myself. Now I could see and understand how the uterus dilated or repair an episiotomy (the incision made to enlarge the vagina for childbirth). I learned to read the strips of paper that unfurled from the monitors that were tracking mother and baby, and with a pang I realized how close to the edge Daniel and I had been when I delivered with my blood pressure so high.

The guiding maxim of our training was "see one, do one," and a third- or fourth-year student who showed willingness and promise had plenty of opportunities to learn by doing. With thirty to forty deliveries a night, every set of eyes and hands was essential. The three or four interns on the floor handled routine deliveries, and even with the help of the family practice and general interns from our programs and other teaching hospitals who cycled through, students were crucial to the operation. The interns on my team were dynamic, teaching at every opportunity and doing it without the caustic edge that was the County hallmark. Even better, the junior and senior residents were women with an equally generous teaching style. They did surgery but without the need for swagger and put-downs. Under them I thrived.

One night I saw the senior and the junior running down the hall with a woman on a gurney, monitoring strips flapping in the breeze. They headed toward the OR for an emergency C-section, but seeing that there was no time, they stopped to do the operation with a local anesthetic—practically in the hallway—and saved the baby's life. It was heroic. Exciting. And undeniably cool.

Not long after, the senior asked me, "How are your knots?" Knots—surgical knots to be precise—were a big deal among the students, and we were encouraged to practice them, both one- and two-handed, whenever we could. Those tiny twists have to be cinched down and fit perfectly against the edges they're binding to prevent bleeding, and it takes time to develop the necessary dexterity. Knots studded the dangling threads on the trashed furniture in the student lounge.

"My knots are good," I told her. I'd taken up stitching and knotting on pillows and stuffed animals after my surgery rotation.

"Great," she said, almost in passing. But a few days later she stopped me. "Come on, Masterson. You want to do a C-section?"

"Really?" I said.

"Whatever you get into I can get you out of," she replied.

So I did it, making an incision two finger widths above the woman's pubic bone, cutting through a fatty layer to a thin, fibrous layer of fascia, then separating and pulling apart the rectus muscles—the "six-pack" muscles of the abdomen. I was working steadily, but time seemed to slow under my focus. Beneath the rectus I could feel the uterus. I pushed the bladder away and, as I had seen the senior do, made a short incision in the uterus, cutting in the shape of a smile. There was no hand-slapping from the senior as she watched, just encouragement and step-by-step coaching. I lengthened the ends of my incision with scissors.

"Okay, Masterson," the senior said. "Reach in, and feel for the baby's head. I'm going to push on top of the uterus while you lift the baby straight out."

I saw its dark hair. We coordinated the tricky pushing and pulling maneuver to remove the baby, clamped the umbilical cord, and handed the baby to a nurse. Then there was the placenta to deliver and all the layers of the abdomen to repack before stitching the torso closed. My knots were close and tight. It was an amazing experience.

"Good job," the senior said. "Now you've done it—go read about it."

The ward was always chaotic, with women up and down the halls screaming and yelling and residents running in and out of rooms with new babies. But it was a well-ordered chaos, and the longer I was there, the more I could make sense of it. It felt like home.

I remember a moment late in my rotation when I'd been up all night checking on women and running from room to room non-stop. Toward the end of the shift, I was sitting with a woman, just the two of us, as the crowning head of her baby pushed toward me. All of a sudden the walls of the room turned a bright yellow, and it was as though something inside me had broken open. It took me a minute to process what was happening. It was sunrise. And I realized I was happy, completely at peace, with a baby sliding into my hands. It filled me up with a joy I still feel. I'd found my calling.

TWENTY

The Prize

Once I knew where I was headed, I kept my eye fixed on the prize: an ob/gyn residency at USC. It was the top-rated program in the country for a reason. There wasn't another in the United States that offered both the intensity of County's crushing workload and the expertise of its staff. The head of the department had written *the* gynecology reference book; the man who'd invented external monitoring for women and fetuses was there, too. My first rotations as a student had left me bone tired, and I still had a long way to go, but if I survived the marathon and got through the residency, I'd be Wonder Woman, ready for anything.

I dutifully made my way through the remaining rotations, each of which seemed to confirm that, for me, nothing could compare to obstetrics. My psychology rotation was in the County psych ward, a secured floor where my office mate and I were taught to use tapping codes to signal each other so we wouldn't open the door to dangerous patients. I wrote case notes on people who paced and stared into the middle distance or offered me their scabs to snack on. I tried to discern the triggers that nudged patients across the flimsy boundary separating the "normal" from the definitely not. The experience gave me great respect for the doctors who can ease those invisible varieties of pain, but I knew I wasn't one of them.

Pediatrics didn't have the urgency of ob/gyn. Orthopedics, and the big jock types on that team, left me cold. They didn't give students much to do, either, which was just fine with me.

The trick was to stay engaged and to keep my face (and hands) in the material that fascinated me the most. As a fourth-year student, I hired on for night shifts in the maternity ward, catching babies. Trained students were entrusted with that task for routine deliveries—and there were many. By the time I graduated, I'd handled between fifty and a hundred. I also signed on for a high-risk pregnancy rotation, which focused on pregnancies like mine, where preeclampsia and its rocketing blood pressure escalate the possibility of complications. We saw women with gallbladder and placenta problems and those whose life-threatening conditions—cancer, say, or an aneurism—had to be factored in. I studied the cases and did my best to be the go-to student on the team. I aced the rotation.

I hoped that a research project would put me over the top for a residency. Through the residents, I heard about an interesting-sounding study, and they steered me to the attending conducting it, Murphy Goodwin. He and another doctor, Richard Paul, were trying to determine if there were a better way to tell if a fetus was in distress in the period right before delivery than scratching its scalp and testing the blood. The scratch test was well established and reliable, but it was invasive and perhaps unnecessary. Dr. Goodwin was gathering data to compare it with another test, called fetal acoustic stimulation, FAS. Rather than scratching the baby, doctors would use a small device, much like the ones designed for artificial larynxes, that emitted a vibrating tone. The procedure was simple: Hold the stimulator against the mother's belly next to the fetus and "buzz" the baby, then measure its heart rate. If the pulse quickened, the baby was healthy.

Both methods had been used at County, and the research would involve going back through the archives and comparing the outcomes of babies who got the scratch test with babies who were simply "buzzed." My job was to look up the blood samplings and other records, gather the numbers, and analyze the data. The doctors would write the paper.

The results were groundbreaking: We found that FAS was just as effective as the scalp blood test, and when we presented the paper, it was the beginning of the end of scratching babies' scalps in the womb. Our work was published in the journal *Obstetrics & Gynecology*.

I applied to residencies and worried through the "match" process, in which students listed their top choices and, through formulas that seemed mysterious to me, were paired with the programs that found them to be the most desirable. At something called the match ceremony in the spring, all the fourth-year students got letters telling them where they'd be spending their residencies, and we were all supposed to open them at the same time. I was too stressed for that. County was the only place I wanted to go, and I wasn't sure what I'd do if I didn't get in. I took the letter to my car to open it so I could have the dignity of falling apart in private if I needed to. Which is how there happened to be shrieks, whoops, and tears of joy filling up a Mustang in the student parking lot on that beautiful April day. I was in.

My mentor from Bishop's, Mrs. Bodenstab, who'd steered me to Mount Holyoke, came up for my graduation ceremony with my mom, and my grandmother flew in from Haynesville. Steve's mom came out, too.

I was looking forward to taking Daniel with me to pick up my diploma. He'd endured a lot of my distraction, especially during my marathon of running from rounds to my piles of data to catching babies on an overnight shift. But he was fussy that day, crying almost constantly. I gathered him up and took him to the stage, thinking he was just overly excited, but when I brought him back, Steve's mom looked at him and said, "Honey, I think there's something wrong with his mouth."

When I took his chin in my hand and gently parted his lips to take a look, I felt like crying. His four front teeth were terribly decayed. We knew that the workers at his day-care center often put him down for naps with juice in his bottle, and we'd asked them not to, but neither Steve nor I had followed up recently. And neither of us had taken a close look at his teeth for quite a while. We'd give them a cursory brushing, dead on our feet, or, just as likely, see him when he was sound asleep.

With the intense workloads of a med student and a fledgling lawyer, something's got to give. We'd let it be Daniel.

The pediatric dentist we saw a few days later had to pull the rotten teeth and fit him for dentures until his next set came in. I'd failed my own baby with my focus on myself. It was time to get my priorities straight.

TWENTY-ONE

Life-and-Death Situations

Daniel had been begging for a trip to the beach, so on a rare weekend off early in my residency, we rolled down the car windows, turned up the radio, and headed west. My mom's friend Joanne was in LA visiting, and she agreed to come along so I'd have a chance to take an occasional break from chasing Daniel. I was dying for some sun—and a chance to see if my boy might have some surfer genes.

It was a gorgeous day, the water gleaming thick and smooth, and the Pacific Coast Highway was clogged, but we spotted a parking lot with a few empty spaces, and I pulled into a turn lane. As we sat waiting, a car traveling at full speed in the opposite direction swerved into my lane, and in a split second it hit us straight on. It came out of nowhere—and I had just enough time to think, "This is it. We're going to die." The impact was crushing, and our white Ford Escort went into a spin. When I came to, someone was at my door, asking if I was all right. I looked back to see about Daniel.

He was crying, but the car seat had held him securely, and he was shaken but not hurt. Joanne was fine, too. But I'd slammed into the windshield and my nose was broken. With police, ambulances, and the wrecks of two cars, we closed down PCH for hours. The drunken driver went to jail, I think, and I went back to County with two black eyes and a cast on my nose. "Hi," I said when I got back. "I'm your new intern." I'd be putting up with stares and jibes for two months, until the cast came off.

I was glad for the two years of rotations I had under my belt. At least I wasn't navigating County for the first time—and I knew exactly what I was in for. Residents who weren't as lucky often got one taste of the tumult and the macho posturing of the place and ran, so most of the people in our program were County survivors, an elite bunch. The intern year had increasing responsibilities, but it still revolved around scut work—keeping the flow of blood work and lab tests going smoothly, being sure that patient records were up to date. We'd all taken our licensing exam before we got our med school diplomas, but we wouldn't be able to prescribe medicine until we'd passed another exam at the end of the year, and we were still being closely vetted.

I had third- and fourth-year med students to run scut for me, and it was my job to train them and scout for talent—some might be valuable as I built my own team in the next few years. Mostly, though, this would be an intense year of taking direction and soaking up as much as I could.

I'd rotate back through the maternity ward, clinics, and The Pit, adding rotations in infertility, oncology, high-risk pregnancy, the neonatal ICU and the pediatric unit. In the maternity ward I was in charge of normal births, talking my own wide-eyed student assistants through the steps of their first deliveries. By the time I'd finished my OB rotation, I'd be expected to have mastered simple C-sections as well. I did mine under the guidance of the senior, and then the junior resident, but when things got crazy, it was hard to hold back from just jumping in to do one with whoever was at hand. I restrained myself. There had been times at the hospital when interns actually did begin assisting each other with the operation, no residents in sight. That was trouble. We still had a lot to learn.

I'd seen an intern get cocky during a C-section and, with hands not quite in position, cut right through the umbilical cord. With the baby and mother now hemorrhaging through the cord, a normal

C-section becomes an emergency; the baby needs to get out as quickly as possible. The senior stepped in for a crash delivery, and neither mom nor baby was harmed. But it was a reminder of how much could go wrong and why we'd be taking years, not just weeks or months, to hone our skills.

We were still working twenty-four-hour shifts that spilled into twenty-eight or thirty. We might be scheduled to go home at seven a.m., but seven could come and go as we did rounds to follow up on the people we'd operated on or sent to the postpartum ward during the night. If a patient came in at the end of the shift and we didn't finish up until noon, it might be four or five before we left. The bathrooms we shared all had showers, which I couldn't believe I'd ever use. But a shower of any kind begins to look attractive when you've been running around sweating for twenty-four hours or longer. Most days I was so tired that even my hair seemed to hurt. I'd get home and ask myself if I'd rather eat or sleep, because I didn't have the energy to do both. I often fell asleep in the middle of a meal.

Shifts like that have since been deemed cruel and unusual, but grueling as they were, I think they made Spartans of us. We gained the confidence that we could do and survive anything. And more concretely, we could watch cases as they unfolded and observe disease processes that take time to evolve. It's a hard experience to replicate unless you give yourself over to following it.

I tried to drive down to see Mom when I could. She'd been healthy since the mastectomy, going on three years by then, but I still wanted to put my arms around her to reassure both of us that she was okay. The time she'd taken off from work to deal with her illness had taken its toll. She'd been forced to leave her job at the EEOC,

I hoped with some kind of retirement package. She wouldn't talk about the specifics.

She'd been taking odd jobs, consulting for companies here and there on workplace issues, and there had been some sort of part-time job for a while. When those dwindled, she took whatever she could get. Her latest position: telephone psychic. "Honey," she said, making light of the whole thing, "if they'll pay me to read tea leaves, I'll read tea leaves."

Christopher was almost a teenager, bright but still struggling with learning difficulties, and Mom kept him in a private school, the only place she thought he could get the attention he needed. A telephone psychic job probably wouldn't cover that. I got the feeling that she was at the end of chasing the lion's tail and might not have the strength anymore to stay ahead of her debts and the schemes she'd always used to pay them.

When I got the cast off my nose, I surprised her with a visit. "There's my doctor!" she said. She looked good, sleeker than before, with a colorful square of silk wrapped around her head. She'd taken to wearing scarves when her hair didn't fully come back after chemo. Wigs, except for special occasions, were too much of a bother, and they were too artificial, she said. She was fine with the way she was.

"I'm glad you're here because I wanted to ask you about this little lump," she said. She guided my hand to a bump on her collar-bone, and when I felt it, I got a sick feeling. In my oncology rotation, we'd looked at the supraclavicular nodes, the lymph nodes that rest on the clavicle. A hard, enlarged node was a classic sign that cancer had spread from another location. This couldn't possibly be good.

"It's probably nothing, Mom," I said. "But you should get it checked out right away, just to be sure."

I was in the middle of a shift at County when her doctor called me with the test results. It was what I'd feared; Mom's cancer had metastasized. The oncologist's best guess was that she had a year—possibly less—to live. "Would you like me to tell her or do you want to do that yourself?" he asked me. My ears were ringing as though I was about to faint, and I leaned against the wall to steady myself. I found some way to say I'd tell her, and I may have hung up in the midst of his condolences. I looked for the junior, the senior, the attending, grabbed the first one and said I was sorry, I had to go. Right away, for an emergency. "Just be sure you're back tomorrow, Masterson," is what I heard. I don't think I explained, just ran, keeping my eyes on the blurring tiles of the floor so no one would see me crying.

I crumpled into my car and sobbed until I was gasping. When I could lift my head and breathe, I called Steve.

"It's Mom," I said, sobbing again.

"What's wrong, are you okay? Honey, what's wrong?" he said.

"I can't drive," I said. "I can't move."

"You're at the hospital? I'll come get you. Just stay there."

I worried over how I'd tell her, what I'd say. But I didn't even have to call. She phoned me, and she knew the answer to "Did you hear anything from the doctor?" from the sound of my voice as I tried to respond. We both cried a while. "Mom," I said finally. "You know, we'll work something out. We always have."

Once you get a diagnosis that grim, you're looking for the pathway to a miracle. I made call after call, searching for clinical trials and studies geared to cancer like hers and found two, one at St. John's Hospital in Santa Monica and the other at USC's Norris Cancer Center. The Norris people were critical of the St. John's approach, but I thought we probably had an even chance with either of them. Mom talked to the St. John's doctors herself, and I sat with her as the Norris docs explained the protocol they'd be using on her. "What do you think, Leese?" she asked me. It wasn't a responsibility I felt I could take. "It's your choice, Mom," I said, rubbing her hand because I didn't want to let it go. She chose Norris, to be close to me, I think. I've wondered ever since if I should've pushed her toward St. John's.

We needed to be together, and the only thing that made sense to me was to move Mom and Christopher up to LA to live with us. Our little place in Glendale wouldn't be nearly large enough, so Steve and I found a two-level house on the Westside that would fit us all, with room for Joanne, who had been taking care of Christopher and now could watch Daniel as well. We couldn't afford to do it, but money was just money. We'd juggle as best we could and figure it out when we had to.

Mom spent a long time looking at schools for Christopher and finally settled on Malibu High, the best public school she could find. There was no use pretending she could afford anything pricier. If Christopher was upset, he wasn't showing it. Like all of us, he seemed to be buoyed up by denial. Mom was the same—only the labels had changed, and maybe the diagnosis was wrong. There was nothing to do but go on.

Having Joanne with us was a blessing—our home had long been the land of spinning plates, with my training and Steve's job and Daniel, and now there was a teenager to get to school and Mom with her rounds and rounds of medical tests and chemo. Joanne ensured that we ate and wore clean clothes and didn't worry about getting Mom and Christopher to where they needed to be. We didn't have the money to pay her, but somehow we did it anyway.

The residency was brutally competitive. With everyone jockeying for better evaluations and spots on the strongest teams, some people took a cutthroat approach: Try to look as good as you can by making the other guy look bad. So it wasn't unusual to come onto a shift and find that the residents before you had left things in a mess—records in the wrong place, messages undelivered, test results unfetched. Nothing that would immediately jeopardize a patient, just enough disarray to ensure that you'd walk into low-level pandemonium. We were all learning to be on our toes 100 percent of the time, looking around the corner and five yards ahead to prevent glitches in the system. And some of our peers seemed to want to see if we could do it after they'd spilled a load of ball bearings on the floor—as if County weren't tough enough on its own.

New rotations reinforced my feeling that I'd found my professional home in obstetrics. Infertility was all about analyzing labs to figure out hormone levels and meds or doing microsurgery to repair infinitesimal tubes. It was completely different from the gritty, large-scale surgery that I found so satisfying—and I hated it. The male clinic was an equally bad fit. As good as my Spanish was, I didn't feel I had the nuances I needed to elicit information sensitively about the size of men's testicles or the details of whether they masturbated.

I tried to run to the hospital to see Mom if I had a break or to sit with her during chemo. Since my residency program was so close, her doctors thought I might want to be involved in her treatment as well. When she needed to get dye into her system before a CAT scan, I started an IV for her after someone else had trouble. When she needed a central line—a catheter that would be used to administer some of her drugs and tests—I observed the surgery. I didn't know if having that sort of access was good or bad. I wanted to know everything about her treatment—she was my mother—but I wanted to look away, too. Most precious to me were the moments

I simply got to be with her after chemo, when the nurses would put her in a bed and let me crawl in beside her.

For the most part she seemed to be doing fine. The treatments would leave her exhausted, and her hair fell out again, but she could still make fun of a nurse's makeup or speculate on the relationships among the medical staff. She was Mom—feisty and inconvenienced by those appointments with toxic chemicals and in full possession of her sense of humor.

I moved into my second year of the residency, one of the major landmarks of the process. I'd angled for a spot on the team of a group of alpha females, sharp women who'd be able to teach me what I needed to learn and defend the work all of us were doing. The second year delivers you into the world of grand rounds, where the second-, third-, and fourth-year residents present their cases for the week and defend their treatment plans, which will then be either annihilated by the attending physicians or praised for their good management of the patients. The burden of grand rounds, also known as M&Ms (for morbidity and mortality conferences) falls on the senior resident, but all of us were on the firing line. The general tenor of grand rounds was caustic. As in battery acid.

By now I was a veteran of C-sections and was assisting with, then performing, more complicated surgeries—repeat C-sections, in which scar tissue became a factor; C-hisses, for C-section hysterectomies in which the uterus is removed after the baby has been delivered. There were deliveries that involved placenta problems and crash C-sections, the adrenaline-fueled emergency operations to keep mothers and babies from dying in high-risk situations. And vacuum deliveries, in which a suction device was attached to the baby's head when a mother couldn't push it out. We even learned to deliver a baby using forceps, just in case we ever needed to do it.

On call in the gyn rotation, we were often on our own. One night we were called to Unit 1, the main County building, to treat a woman who had a ruptured abscess on her fallopian tubes. My senior and I drove up to the ER and started opening the woman up, but when we looked into the abdomen, we couldn't see discrete organs—everything looked like mush. The attending didn't want to get out of bed and come over, so the senior tried to describe the mush over the phone. It was a horrible feeling, knowing how little time we had and how disoriented we were. On another night we opened an abdomen full of blood and had to try to locate the source of the bleeding guided only by the voice of an attending on the phone who couldn't see the body in front of us. It was terrifying.

The patients did amazingly well. County's hands-on approach to medical training—"see one, do one"—felt ridiculously risky when we were in the thick of a complication we'd never encountered before. Yet in the vast majority of cases, we all made it through— the women on the table as well as the rattled apprentices who were frantically trying to save them. And in working to resolve the crises in front of us, so often with no attending beside us, we learned to trust that we could handle whatever County, or hell, threw at us.

TWENTY-TWO

Without Her

When I went to visit Mom for one of her chemo sessions during the summer, she was standing outside the building waiting for me. "I'm done," she said. "I can't do this anymore."

I clicked into doctor mode. "You can't be done, Mom," I said. "I know you may not feel great now, but we're getting results. You'll see."

She looked exhausted. "Leese, I just can't." Her gaze slipped from mine, and she seemed small and frail, even as she stood solidly in front of me.

"Mom, come on, let's go in. You've got to keep going." I felt pushy and selfish and desperate. I needed her to give the treatments all she had, and for me she tried. Every once in a while, though, she'd want to shoo away my denial and talk about death. I just couldn't let her. A lifetime's worth of "We'll get through *this*, too" ran interference between the reality of her illness and the part of me that might be able to acknowledge it. But we did have one small moment in the car toward the end of the summer. She'd begun to lose her wit, her sense of humor, and as I drove I remember thinking, "This is not Mom—it's not her."

As if she'd sensed an opening, she quietly told me, "The worst part of this is how much I'm going to miss you, honey."

I couldn't let her words in right then. "Oh, Jesus, Mom," I said. "That's not going to happen." I wished either of us had it in us to turn on the radio just one more time and sing.

As we closed in on the one-year mark, the date that had been looming for so long, I began to think we'd been living under the oh-so-frightening shadow of a garden gnome, not the grim reaper. "They're full of crap, those doctors," I told Steve. "She's so much better than they said."

Just two weeks later, right before Halloween, I had the day off, and we'd made a play date with one of Daniel's friends, who was coming over to carve pumpkins. We were laughing and planning our jack-o'-lanterns in the kitchen when I thought to check on Mom. She was sitting in the dining room trying to eat, but she couldn't keep a grip on her spoon. I was scared for her. Disoriented and weak, she was fading.

I asked Joanne to watch the kids, and Mom and I headed for the hospital. I was supposed to be on call with my team, and when I phoned to let them know what had happened, all they could say was, "So when are you coming back?"

"If my mother dies soon, I'll be back soon," I said. "If not, it'll be later."

Mom lost consciousness hours after we arrived. In my oncology rotation we'd watched patients move through their final days, organs shutting down one by one, and I knew that must be happening now. The cancer had spread to her liver, which could no longer detoxify her body, and her kidneys were slowing down as well. I stayed in her room, sitting by her bed and calling my advisor to brainstorm about anything we could do to help her. With Mom in a coma, the nurses pushed me hard to take her off life support. One of them was sure that she'd heard Mom ask not to be resuscitated, but I knew she was wrong, and I battled with the staff to make sure we did everything possible to keep her alive.

One of my great comforts was my grandmother, who came to be with us. She still blamed herself for not insisting that Mom have a mastectomy earlier, though we both knew that neither of us could've saved her. Grandma stayed beside me, waiting and praying. I watched the tests and MRIs and monitors, all of them showing the slow winding down of Mom's systems. I could see it happening, but I couldn't see it at all. This was my deepest fear, the plane crash I had dreamed of so often as a child—but I'd wake from this nightmare, I was certain, and she'd be there. I denied and argued and bargained with all my might, trying to push death away.

For long hours I held her hand and rubbed it. I'd been eating, sleeping, and showering in her room, my only respite coming from a friend at County, who called me every day to tell me a joke. For a couple of minutes, we'd laugh, and I'd begin to feel like myself. But by the fourth day, exhaustion wearing down my defenses, I could finally let in the reality of losing her. "You can't die on me now, Mom," I told her, tears coming at last. "Please, Mom. Come back to me."

Her eyes fluttered open as I sobbed. The sound of my crying must have penetrated some deep place, and she looked at me concerned, saying, "Lisa, what's wrong?"

It was as though she'd just awakened from a nap, and she was as lucid as she'd ever been.

Christopher had been coming to visit after school, never staying more than a few minutes. He didn't quite get what was going on, even though I tried to tell him. But when Mom came back, she drew him close for a chat, insisting on good-byes even though they seemed premature now that everything had changed. I knew they had. We'd find a new treatment—I was sure of it.

"Honey, you know it's going to be okay," she told me. "You be strong for me, all right? And your brother—don't you throw him out like the garbage." She flashed a smile, but there was steel behind it. "You take good care of Christopher."

With Mom seeming better, Grandma flew back to Haynesville to take care of Grandpa. But Steve had a premonition, and he wouldn't let me stay in the hospital alone. When he got to the room that evening, Mom was sleeping, her breathing shallow and noisy—that "death rattle" I'd heard on the oncology wards. I'd been listening to that sound night after night, but it seemed more pronounced now, and when we woke in the morning, she was still breathing that way, unresponsive when we tried to rouse her. When she came around again, I could hear her repeating something, but I couldn't make out the words.

"Water? Did she say she wants some water, Steve?" I asked him.

"No, honey," he said softly. "She's saying, 'I love you.'"

Mom blinked at me one last time, and then her breathing stopped.

The monitors squealed, and I buzzed for the nurses and called the code. The staff was racing her to the ICU just as my uncles Almer and Don walked toward the room. I was beside Mom in the ICU when she coded again. This time she wouldn't come back.

I'd pronounced patients dead on the oncology ward and had the profound experience of seeing families weep for their loved ones. Now I was one of them, screaming and wailing so inconsolably that the doctors suggested sedation. I felt as though my heart—the purest, most loving part of me—had been ripped from my being. I could scarcely bear the pain. It didn't make sense. I'd saved all those babies—how was it possible I couldn't save her?

Leaving the hospital without my mom was one of the hardest things I've ever done. I didn't know how the world could go on, but I found that it tugged me along, or tried to, as it kept turning. I went home to bed, pulled the shades, and refused to eat. I lay in the darkness, hoping it would simply snuff out any light in me and let me die in peace. But there were funerals to attend to, two of them—one in San Diego, one in Haynesville. I pulled on my clothes, for the first time in days, for the drive to San Diego. I was numb with grief, but the priest wanted me to say something. It was a mistake. I stumbled up to the pulpit and unleashed the anger I felt over losing Mom so soon. It came out in the form of an attack on the friends and family who'd gathered to pay their respects. "Why are you here?" I shouted. "You don't even know this woman, how wonderful she was. She was everything to me. I'm glad you came, but it's too late. You didn't care about her!"

Tears overtook me before I could go on, and the priest gently tried to recover, reassuring me that "we all loved her."

My grandmother was a healing presence for me in Haynesville, and our deep connection soothed me. There was an open casket at the funeral home, and I was supposed to join the mourners viewing Mom's body, but that was more than I could bear. I started to go in but froze in the doorway and asked to be taken home. The body was out again at the service in Grandma and Grandpa's church, which was filled with friends and family who'd known Mom when she was Baby Rae, the smart little girl on Grandma's hip. I kept my eyes on Grandma or the floor and pretended the casket was a piece of furniture. I knew Mom, and whatever was in the casket wasn't her.

My father came with his family, and the words I wanted to say right then blasted through my mind: "Get out of my face!" was the kindest of them. I was an angry kid again, thinking, "I'm not going to be your friend now. You will never be anything to me! If I was loyal to Mom in her life, you can be sure I'll be loyal to her now." Thank God all I could get out was "Hello." With Mom gone

I wanted scorched earth around me, but at least in Haynesville my better angels kept me quiet.

At my grandparents' cemetery plot, the casket was lowered into the ground and cement was poured over the top, the finality of it so heavy that I could feel it in my chest. Grandma handed Christopher and me knobs from the casket to keep. Christopher, though his life would change far more than mine, seemed less traumatized that I was, and he was eating, playing with his cousins—functioning. I clearly was not. Back home, I crawled back into bed and refused to get up.

Steve was beside himself as days passed and I hardly moved. He didn't know if he should take me to a doctor or try to find someone else to intervene. He asked my school advisors to call me, and I think they all talked about whether I'd need to be hospitalized if I didn't start eating and making some small move toward trying to stay alive. I wanted nothing more than to disappear. This time there was no Mom to pull me back.

But a couple of weeks into my isolation, the door to my room pushed open and my son Daniel stood in the light that spilled in from the hallway. "Mommy," my four-year-old said, "I need you to be my mommy again."

I blinked hard, startled, and something in me struggled to sit up. I held out my arms, and Daniel ran to me. "Oh, honey," I said, rubbing my face into his soft hair, "I'm here." I could've held him forever, but after nestling into me, he squirmed out of my grip. "Mommy, I'm hungry," he said. "Let's eat."

I've never felt closer to my son than I felt then, and that closeness has never faded. It's the unbreakable, irreplaceable bond that reaches from my grandmother to my mother to me and now to him—and to all the mothers and children I treat. When I work to save a baby or ensure that a mother will live to care for her children, I'm blowing on the ember of love that will let them save each other and keep them moving through life together. It's my way of thanking Mom and the tiny, precious boy who gave me a reason to go on when she was gone.

The land of the living was fractured when I returned. Christopher was in our care, and he struggled against Steve and me now that we were his guardians. He ran away to friends' houses, and I sent Steve out repeatedly to find him. We met with his teachers and tried to reassure him that he'd be all right with us, that we were family. But he'd just lost his mother, and like a younger, uncensored version of me, he let his pain and anger blast out. He wasn't having any of us. Finally, I called Emmett to see if he would be willing to take in his son, and to our eternal gratitude he agreed. Steve took Christopher the same day on a plane to Seattle, and Emmett and his wife became the family my brother needed until he graduated a couple of years later and joined the Marines.

By now three months had passed since I left my team at the hospital, and when I was finally ready to go back, there was no easy reentry. The junior and senior on my team never really expressed any sympathy, just irritation that I'd left them in the lurch. We'd all taken a first step into the world of doctoring by learning to deal dispassionately with injury and disease, putting our work before our emotions. It was too early in the process, probably, to expect compassion from people who were learning to survive County by pushing their feelings away. If you couldn't do that, the pain might pull you under. Still, I was stung. At every turn I could feel people sizing up my wounds and asking, "Is she really going to make it now?" I knew I had to get back on track for my mom and my son, and I answered the doubts with defiance. If my fellow doctors-to-be couldn't offer up any support, I'd be the badass doctor who didn't need it.

I became a rebel, with bracelets on my arm and a "don't mess with me" attitude. We all wore clogs, but now mine had stiletto heels. The nurses knew when I was on duty in The Pit: I was the one blasting Peter Gabriel's "Red Rain" as I operated. I was bleeding, the patients were bleeding—it was my cri de coeur in those difficult months. Damn it, I was going to survive!

My "spiked and pierced" attitude didn't endear me to anyone. As I finished that second year of residency, my team announced that they were dumping me. That meant I went into my third year on a team of "leftovers," people who hadn't managed to cement relationships with the teams they wanted. I'd gone from the best team to one led by a weak senior who got crushed at grand rounds (also called "stats" for the statistics we presented about our patients' conditions). The abuse our senior took there filtered down to the rest of the team, and a bad performance at stats meant heaps of blame for the second-year resident and me. It only made me want to be harder and smarter.

There were other challenges. A crazy kind of sexual tension erupted among some of the male staff and residents I dealt with. Guys would masturbate loudly on the bunk above me when I was trying to rest in one of our call rooms, or they'd make advances. It felt like more of the macho County hazing, and it reached its extreme when one of my attendings took me aside and told me, "If you sleep with me, I'll tell you the director's favorite cigars and help you get them."

"Are you for real?" I said, walking away. I didn't have time for those kind of games. Some women might've complained or sued, but I needed to get on with things. I was already running behind,

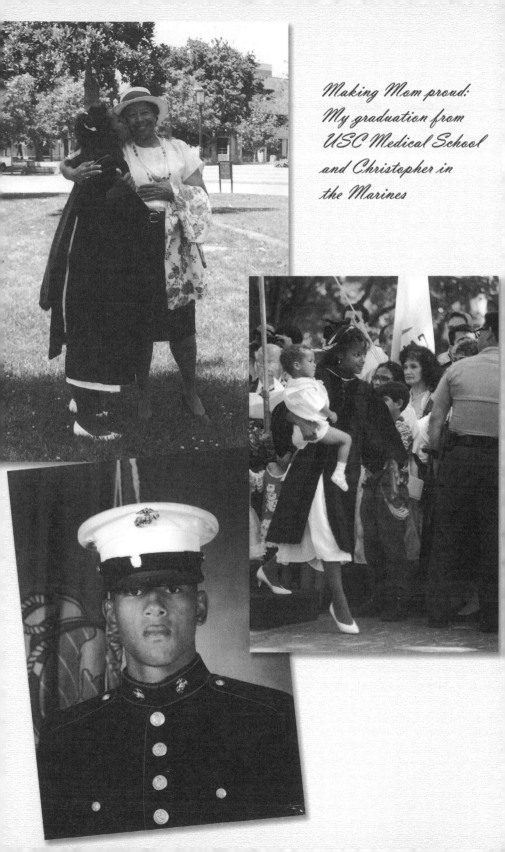

Making Mom proud:
My graduation from
USC Medical School
and Christopher in
the Marines

and the school wasn't going to forgive me the time I'd missed. I'd have another three months of rotations tacked on to my last year.

A couple of friends, Christina and Scanlon, kept me sane. Chris and I had the kind of bond that comes from working side by side under pressure. We had the odd experience of touching inside a patient when Chris was pushing a baby's head up during a C-section so I could pull the baby out of the incision. Making that kind of contact is rare, and it stuck with us, that shared experience. She and Scanlon ran interference if they saw a male attending getting out of line with me, and they talked me into going out occasionally after a shift to let off steam.

My real salvation, though, came in the form of Joanne, a urology fellow I'd met during one of my rotations, who took me out for coffee and threw me a lifeline. "I know you have a lot of people looking at you and expecting you to fail," Joanne told me. "You don't deserve that, and I'm going to help you." Specifically, she offered to tutor me in the kind of thinking that would let me master grand rounds. She'd sit with me and help me work through the best way to describe and explain cases.

I'd set myself up to take on the world by myself, but I soaked up her help and learned a way of organizing and presenting my week's statistics and cases that let me see them through the eyes of the attendings who would be lobbing queries about them. I practiced with her and on my own, watching my team's senior resident crumble during stats but mentally trying out my own alternate presentations. And when the attendings threw me an occasional question, I tried out our strategy.

The key, she said, was thinking ahead. As a senior I'd be analyzing the cases our team was handling and the treatment I'd been directing. The drill was that I'd make a list of our patients, the treatments we'd tried, and the outcomes, typing it up and getting it in by Wednesday so the attendings would have handouts to look at for grand rounds on Friday. They'd look through the list, ask about Patient X or Y, and grill me about what we'd done. Joanne showed me that I could write up the information to elicit certain questions and anticipate the responses we'd get. "There's no way they're not going to ask you about this," she'd say, pointing to a particular spot in my notes, "because it's so pertinent to the case." She didn't tell me what to say, she taught me how to see the big picture and think ahead in ways that all those years of "pimping" from the attendings had not. The gift she gave me was priceless, and it serves me to this day.

When I got to my final year, and fielded grand rounds alone for the first time, I was ready.

Twenty-three

Call Me Dr. Masterson

I turned heads at stats. No longer was I the "outsider who might not make it"—people said I did some of the best grand rounds in years. I could get to the heart of a case, anticipate questions, and essentially look at my patients and decisions just as the attendings would; that is, I could think like a doctor. It was intimidating to be in the hot seat, directing the care of so many patients, but I trusted myself. It was as though a million random bits of knowledge and experience had pulled themselves into a coherent picture, and my hands and eyes and mind finally knew how to connect with the clarity that brings healing. I was becoming the physician I wanted to be.

Losing Mom had given me the additional gift of letting me feel how the illness or death of a mother or child rippled through families and communities. If I'd started out wanting to master technical skills, now I understood from the inside what it meant to be able to offer comfort, or a chance at a longer life.

I ached to talk to Mom. She'd believed in me no matter what, and finally, here I was, a young black woman holding her own in the macho old boys' club of County. I could feel her laughing at the surprise on their faces—and wrapping me up in her pride.

When you're good, people want to jump onto your team, and I was able to choose the best of the junior and second-year residents to work with me. With most procedures in their competent hands,

I could not only stay on top of cases but even enjoy the process. We were still working shifts that went on for days, and we were among the last to face the worst of County's intensity. It's a different place now, a change that began in earnest when private doctors began to accept MediCal payments, and suddenly, many of the poor who'd flocked to our teeming public hospital could choose their own physicians. Surviving the onslaught of the old days is a mark of honor for classes like mine, and I know the process tempered us. We're harder, perhaps, than some of the doctors who've followed us. But we're also strong—and resilient.

In that last training year, I was still the rebel in stiletto clogs— and also the control freak I'd always been, the "give it 110 percent" girl. I had my hands on everything, and unlike some of the more relaxed senior residents, I was always calling my team to find out what was going on or dropping in for surprise rounds. Part of my job was handling the most complicated surgeries—vaginal hysterectomies, C-section hysterectomies, and women's third or fourth C-sections. It gave me a lot of pleasure, this hard-won proficiency at running my team and caring for patients, especially when I knew people expected me to fail.

I didn't have a clear picture of what I wanted to do when my residency was done. "It's sick," I told my mentor, "but I like grand rounds—preparing and being prepared, figuring out what I'll be asked, presenting the cases. I could see myself doing something educational." I didn't know what that might be, maybe something in public health, or teaching in a residency program. Private practice, being my own boss, was appealing, too. I glimpsed yet another possibility when I was taking care of one of the mundane tasks that fell to seniors—booking speakers for grand rounds. Every week, after the attendings were done grilling and flaying our teams of residents, we'd regroup by listening to lectures. The idea was that we'd get a sense of the wider world of medicine, maybe even meet someone who'd inspire us. One of the people I brought in was a gynecological oncologist who volunteered his services at clinics in underserved regions of Asia and Africa. A friend had recommended him, and I'd scheduled him casually, figuring he'd be interesting. But afterward, I couldn't stop thinking about the stories he told of people dying for want of the cheapest, simplest supplies—sutures!—or basic care. I took his card and put it where I wouldn't lose it.

There was no time off for good behavior in my program, even for someone at the top of her game. I had missed three months to attend to Mom, and good performance or no, I'd have to stay on after everyone else graduated to make up rotations. Rumors spread about why I was still there. Mostly, people assumed that I'd failed something, but my only "failing" was that my mom had died. It was painful to see my class graduate without me. How odd that I'd always been ahead of them, but now I was being left behind. I spent my last months at County running a clinic, and without the pressure of surgery, it was simple. But my next move would be extremely tough: My classmates had snapped up every available placement. I'd be a freshly minted doctor with no job and a lot of debt.

No ceremony awaited me when I was done—just my diploma. I was invited to attend a graduation with the next class, months later, but that seemed pointless. So my last day at the hospital was just another day. When I walked out the doors, I felt like a person who'd just been released from prison—and I didn't quite know what to do, or how I'd go through life outside the pressure cooker that was County. It had taken years to get to know the staff, the maze of a hospital and the art and disciplines of functioning in that high-stress environment. Now I was free to choose something new.

It was paralyzing at first. I could go for a fellowship in a specialty such as infertility or maternal/fetal medicine, but I didn't want to be, say, a consultant on high-risk pregnancies. That would mean giving up delivering babies. Infertility work would put me back behind the microscope looking at sperm. I didn't want to give up any of the variety and challenges of being an ob/gyn. So, armed with a stack of recommendations from my attendings, I began to see what kind of work I could drum up. The card I'd saved from Leo Lagasse, the globe-traveling oncologist caught my eye—I felt drawn to the relief work he was doing—and I called him to see if he had advice or leads. As a matter of fact, he said, he had trips planned to Africa and the Philippines. Did I want to go? He didn't have the funds to cover my accommodations in Africa, but if I could pay my way to the Philippines, he'd take care of my food and lodging.

Steve could see the look in my eye, and even though the expense would be a strain, he said he thought we could manage a plane ticket. So I went to help treat women who'd had abnormal Pap smears. It was my first trip abroad.

The doctor had raised money for the clinic where we were operating, so we were blessed with decent equipment and the luxury of air-conditioning. But when I went to look at the obstetrics side of the operation, I was struck by the run-down facilities. I didn't think there could be a place worse than The Pit, but I'd come face to face with it. In the labor rooms three or four women crowded into a single bed, with no fetal monitors or pain medication. And when it was time to deliver, residents would walk women over to a huge room where they'd climb onto hard metal tables covered with dried blood to push their babies—many of them dead—into the world. Here, women we could've saved at County often died from postpartum hemorrhaging. I knew the cancer surgery we'd come to do was vital, but when I heard families wailing because they'd lost a baby or mother who should have survived, I was struck to my core.

"This just shouldn't be," a voice in my head kept repeating. I only stayed a week, but I knew I needed to do more. This was work that I'd return to as soon as I could. Right now, though, I needed a job.

I put out feelers at hospitals around Los Angeles and was lucky enough to meet Dr. Gail Jackson, a popular ob/gyn with a busy practice at Cedars Sinai. Dr. Jackson was a light-skinned black woman with great business savvy and a directness and sense of humor that reminded me of my mom's. She promised to work my tail off, but in return she'd show me how to navigate the world of a private practice in a very political hospital and how to thrive in an HMO world. We were a good fit personality-wise, with the same work ethic. And she understood what it was like to balance home life with a career—as the single mother of a teenager, she didn't mind seeing Daniel waiting in the office for me or being flexible about my schedule as long as we got the work done and took care of our patients.

Dr. Jackson knew a good thing when she saw it, and she scheduled me for as many as forty or fifty appointments a day. The reality of the HMO world is that many patients get just ten or twelve minutes of a doctor's attention, and if a quick checkup is all that's needed, that's what's offered. A patient with serious concerns or complications would naturally get more time, but for routine visits I'd have to cut off casual conversations about movies and boyfriends—unless a woman was telling me about a lifestyle choice that put her in danger, something like having unprotected sex.

Even with those efficiencies, I'd often find that I'd been double-booked, so patients had to wait to see me, though I was theoretically right on schedule. We worked an eight-hour day, but both of us were on call with our own patients, and sheer numbers meant that there would sometimes be a lot of babies arriving at the same time. On my busiest night I delivered nine, an ordinary shift at County but fairly remarkable for a private practice.

Grueling as the pace might've seemed, it felt almost luxurious to me. My patients were all getting good prenatal care, all of them spoke English, and it was rare to see the devastating complications that come when an emergency brings a woman in for the first doctor's visit of her pregnancy. I got close to my moms-to-be in the months before delivery, and many became friends. My life was definitely better, starting with basics, such as having time to eat and sleep. I gained a lot of weight in that first year because instead of running all over a huge hospital, I was mostly in our offices, and when drug reps brought in lunch, I actually sat down to enjoy it.

I still had my rough rebel edges at first, but Dr. Jackson was full of pragmatic advice. "If you're going to work with men in our profession," she'd say, "you have to back off a little." At County I had grown accustomed to confronting men who challenged me. As far as I could tell, competing with them was the only way to survive. At Cedars, though, that aggressiveness wasn't serving me.

"You can use that 'get in their faces' approach," Gail told me, "but it's not going to work here." What worked with our male colleagues, she said, was to just "rub their bellies and pat their heads and get what you want in a different way."

Respect was hard to come by, but she insisted on it. "Notice how the nurses and patients don't call you 'doctor,'" she observed one day. I'd noticed all right—it drove me crazy that practically any male in the place was addressed as "doctor," but people on every level pushed to address me by my first name. I didn't know if it had to do with my age, my race, my gender, or some combination, but no matter what I did, I was "Lisa." Dr. Jackson would correct anyone she heard using just my first name, and she was adamant:

"Don't succumb to that," she told me. "Anyone with respect will change what they call you if you ask, but people seem to be short on that. They just don't want to give you the title."

She fought that battle herself, and I loved the way she'd tell people, "I'm hard of hearing and I'm used to hearing the word 'doctor' before my name." It seemed to work. I also learned to say, again and again, "Please, call me Dr. Masterson, or if you prefer, call me Dr. Lisa." Call me anything you want, I wanted to say, just be sure you call me "doctor" first.

Dr. Jackson kept a smile on her face even when the politics of the HMO and hospital rankled and she had to fight to keep patients that someone wanted to siphon away. Her practice blossomed. And as I soaked up her pragmatic nurturing, I began to learn something that had come naturally to Mom but had always been a little foreign to me: charm.

Twenty-four

I Love Lucy

I didn't know how to relax. At work my mind was still ever vigilant, looking and anticipating, always working. County, with its crisis-a-minute pace, was receding into the past, but I was still trip-wired. I was so used to handling endless tasks daily that I think I almost reflexively created more activity for myself once I began practicing. That's the only way I can explain how, within just a few months, I found myself falling into a branching series of unexpected ventures.

Our office was on the west side of Los Angeles, and it was common for us to see women who worked in the entertainment business. Actresses, writers, and producers—along with all those small names you see when the movie credits roll—need physicians, and soon I was getting a window into the industry from my patients. One of them, who produced a local TV news program, stuck her head back in the door as she was leaving an appointment and said, "You know, I've been thinking. You'd probably be good on a segment I'm doing on women's health. Why don't you call me, and we can talk about it." She pulled out her card and said, "Let's touch base this week, okay? I'm liking this idea."

We worked out the details, and I made my way over to the studio, where someone patted some powder on my face. The producer reviewed the topic I'd be answering questions about—it was one of the common ones, fibroids or hormones—introduced me to the program's host, and set me in front of the camera. I was nervous walking in, but I knew my stuff. And no one, I told myself, would ever be able to grill me the way I'd been grilled at County. Indeed, the interview, friendly and informal, was a breeze compared with the firing-squad approach I was used to from grand rounds.

When I saw myself on tape, I thought I'd done all right. So did my patient. She booked me for another segment, and another, and before I knew it, I was regularly using my pre- and postappointment hours to tape segments for a women's health program, then a teen program on Fox. The basic approach I'd learned for organizing my thoughts and prompting people to ask me the questions I wanted them to ask served me well, and it went a long way toward putting me at ease. It was funny; I'd had trouble back when I was trying out for TV and commercial roles in college because people said I didn't seem comfortable in my own skin. Now I knew what that comfort was about for me: being my actual self, sharing my own real expertise.

I loved the way a single appearance, even on a local TV show, could reach exponentially more people with a health message than I'd ever see one on one in an office. I hadn't imagined anything like this when I'd thought about doing health education, but why not, I thought. It was working.

I'm not sure how high the bar was for those early appearances. There was no coaching, and I think that at first people were happy simply because I didn't lapse into jargon or tighten up when someone wanted to talk about sex. It was a plus that I seemed to be enjoying myself, whatever the topic.

The more segments I did, the more calls I got, and after a while my media exposure gave me the confidence to consider opening my own practice and running it the way I imagined, with all the bells and whistles I knew would elevate the standard of care and comfort for both the women who came in and me. Some things, such as an ultrasound machine, I thought of as necessities. Others, such as tables that could easily move a patient into different positions, were just touches I thought could make a positive difference. The thing was, I wanted to be able to customize equipment and protocols for treatment myself. So when I heard about a doctor who was looking for someone to take over his practice, I went to talk with him. When he said he'd let me try things out, working half time at first, I jumped at the chance. The contrast was striking. The new practice had a preferred-provider arrangement with insurance companies, and our patients there often paid us cash. We could afford to make appointments longer, and I had the feeling that I was really getting to know the women who came in.

I was also getting to know the moms at Daniel's school in Bel Air, an enclave of affluent families and people in the entertainment business. When the women I met there wondered if they and their friends might come to the office, I liked being able to say yes and invite them to my own practice. I liked the idea of having more control over my own schedule, too. With media calls coming in thick and fast, that was going to be important.

Finally, after a hectic year of working in both offices, I was able to jump into a practice of my own. A doctor was selling hers, and I worked out an arrangement with a third doctor who would buy it and pay me to work there. Once things were up and running, and I was pulling in more of my own patients, I'd begin making payments toward the price of the practice. With no real financial strain, I was on my own.

I couldn't make my mind stop cranking out ideas, most having to do with meeting needs that I saw in the office day after day. Young moms with tween girls—not to mention the moms from Daniel's school—were starting to ask me how to talk to their kids about sex and puberty. They didn't want to copy their parents' approach—which tended to be either "ignore it" or "hand 'em a pamphlet and a pad"—but they didn't know how to do better.

Synapses started firing in my brain. What if we could get kids solid information about their bodies before they were too intimidated to ask questions? One thing I knew from seeing patients and reading the literature was that the women who came in with STDs almost uniformly had a poor self-image. But if you could reach them early, and give them the information to feel confident about their bodies, you could go a long way toward solving that problem—and others, such as an unwanted pregnancy.

I made an appointment with the principal of Daniel's school, a man I'd met years ago when my madrigal group from Bishop's sang there. We both liked the idea of doing health education for the fourth, fifth, and sixth graders that would cover the way the body changes in adolescence and segue into sex education for the older kids. I developed a curriculum, which we refined and presented to the parents, and to our surprise it was met with enthusiasm—everyone loved it. I'd planned to talk just to the girls, because I didn't want to embarrass Daniel—the last thing he needed, I thought, was for his mom to show up in his classroom talking about penises. But after I did the first presentation to the fourth-grade girls, he asked me, "Why don't you teach a boys' class?" I was joyfully dumbfounded, but I still taught only the girls until he graduated.

I loved the kids. Fresh and young and completely uninhibited, they asked all kinds of questions we didn't anticipate. They were fascinated with tampons. How do they get in there? Will they get stuck? And when we talked about hormonal changes that would alter their chemistry and body odors, they'd ask things like, "Why do we need to smell?" Unlike older kids, they had no preconceived ideas, and they asked questions because they were genuinely curious, not to shock each other or shut each other down. I had a chance to follow the same bunch of kids over three years, and each spring I met them with a slightly different curriculum and message. The school found a video we could show, and the program was so popular that other private schools also invited me to come in to present it. By the time Daniel graduated, my practice had grown too busy to let me continue teaching the classes, but the school kept my curriculum. I never heard a single complaint from a parent.

Steve would just shake his head when I got carried away with an idea. And I had lots of them. Teaching the classes, and seeing tween girls in my practice, made me wish we had something we could give girls for that big rite of passage, their first period. I remembered well how I'd gotten mine on the bus and didn't want to talk to my mom about it. But what if Mom had been able to give me something pretty, something feminine to say, "It's okay. Welcome to womanhood." My imagination carried me away. There was one tampon kit on the market, but it was corduroy and crass—a guy must've designed it, I thought. I had something different in mind— a silky bag that would hold a pad or a tampon, a towelette, a change of underwear, and a wheel in bright colors that you could use to predict your period. I'd put in a short booklet about what to expect, what to do for cramps and PMS. And there would even be a piece of chocolate. I'd call it the B'Cool Kit.

Some people would've let it go at that—let the fantasy stay a fantasy—but I am probably the biggest *I Love Lucy* fan of all time, and I sprang into action. The person who did my makeup for one of the TV shows had a makeup bag I liked, and I got the name of the manufacturer. They could make the bag for my kit—but only if I got three thousand. I ordered three thousand pink bags. Then I'd need my PMS/period wheel. Drug companies hand out pregnancy wheels, a similar concept, to doctors, so I called the number on one of the wheels and got a price. They could design and make a period wheel for me, but the smallest order was five thousand. They'd give me a deal on pregnancy wheels as well, if I had some done at the same time. So I got five thousand of each. I ordered chocolate mints. Assembled the other pieces. Put my booklet together. And I started handing out the bags. If you happen to need one, I still have a lot on hand. Several hundred probably would've been plenty for my purposes. I made a lifetime supply.

While I was at it, I decided to put together a book with my sex-education lessons for high school kids. I gathered my notes, found a writer to help me organize them, and got some people in the graphics department at Cedars to do cartoons and bind everything up. This time I went for a smaller scale—we created just fifty books—but I still use them for presentations, and kids still respond to the humorous approach.

I have a tendency to get obsessive when I get interested in solving a problem, especially one that has to do with health. I set things in motion, and the "chocolates" start rushing down the conveyor belt, sometimes faster than I can handle them. But I can't think of a better way to find out what's possible—though Steve might say that there must be cheaper ones.

I'd thought, after my Mom died, that I was done with funerals for a while. But I was just a year into working with Dr. Jackson when my grandfather had a massive heart attack while visiting friends. Grandpa had been the soul of his community, and the funeral, held in the church he'd raised and been such a part of, was intensely emotional. We gathered at the grave under big white tents and wept as they lowered him into the ground. He was only in his seventies, and all of us had assumed he'd live to one hundred.

Grandma was never the same after that. I spoke to her often by phone, and my uncle Don moved to Haynesville to be near her, but when I went down to visit, I saw that she was wasting away. Depression and diabetes were taking her over. The little hospital in Haynesville couldn't seem to get things under control, so I rode with her in an ambulance to a hospital in Shreveport, where she seemed to improve. But back home, she declined again, and over the next couple of years, her health was tenuous at best. I was startled, but perhaps not surprised, when I got a call from my uncle saying that Grandma was in the Haynesville hospital again, and this time they thought she was dying.

Grandma was unconscious in the ICU when I arrived, and the doctors urged me to take her off all life support. "It's not going to be my call," I told them. "It's her decision to make." I stayed for four days, sleeping in a hospital room down the hall, watching movies on a computer with my uncle, and sitting with Grandma, talking to her and rubbing lotion into her hands, just as I'd done with Mom. She hadn't been speaking clearly when she arrived at the hospital, my uncle told me, and she'd had trouble moving half of her body, but the doctors weren't certain if she'd had a stroke or if her diabetes had progressed and was causing the problems. I didn't know if we'd have a chance to find out—I just wanted to be able to talk to her one more time. Finally, on the fourth day of my visit, she amazed us all by opening her eyes, looking into mine, and saying, "Lisa?"

I had to leave the next day to do an interview with *Good Morning America*, and I'd worried that she wouldn't come around before I left. But by some miracle we were able to talk one last time—about Mom and me and Daniel—and I got to tell her how much I loved her. It was one of the great blessings of my life. She'd been another mother to me, especially after Mom died, and she was one of the few people in my life who knew how far I'd come from Haynesville. Even with Steve and Daniel and my uncles, I felt very alone in the world when she was gone. I could hardly bear to see another grave. I didn't have any more tears.

Twenty-five

Butterflies and Oprah

The phone rang often with calls from producers and bookers for TV shows. I was intrigued to hear about *The Other Half*, a talk show on NBC that aspired to be the male equivalent of *The View*. Dick Clark was its host, and the panel it pulled together to chat about the issues of the day included Danny Bonaduce, the former child star. The producers invited me to answer questions about women's health and to give a woman's perspective, and because I got on well with the hosts, they invited me fairly regularly. A high point was the day David Cassidy, one of Bonaduce's costars on *The Partridge Family*, dropped by the show. I'd had a Partridge Family lunchbox as a kid, and for a moment or two, I was an eight-year-old bouncing with the crazy excitement of "It's them!"

The show only lasted a few years, but it was a great training ground for me. One of the producers was something of a perfectionist, and she became the first person to give me any real direction. Rather than simply letting me walk on and do my thing, she wanted to know what I was going to say, and then she wanted me to practice. "Why don't you say/do/emphasize this," was her common refrain. It drove me crazy, but I smiled and did my part her way, one more time—take after take. *The Other Half* was my first talk show, a completely different atmosphere from the news interviews I'd done, and over time I began to master what was needed: high energy, a lot more projection, succinct sound bites.

With more polish came different kinds of opportunities. I became a spokesperson for Johnson & Johnson and made pilots for a couple of health-related shows that didn't get picked up. I was a regular guest on *Berman and Berman*, a Discovery Health show hosted by a pair of doctor sisters who discussed women's health and sexuality, and a program called *What Should You Do?* frequently asked me to be one of the medical experts answering the title question in all sorts of life-threatening scenarios. I was amazed and humbled to think about how many people I could reach with these appearances. I could talk about health and self-esteem and sexuality, and there was a good chance millions of people would get good information.

All of this came about, I'm certain, because I'd never lost touch with my mom's maxim: "Nothing beats a winner but a try." In every part of my life, my typical answer to the strange ideas and opportunities that fell onto my path was, "Sure I've never done it before. But what have I got to lose?" I can't say I had a Zen attitude and "beginner's mind"—I don't like fumbling or failing—but I did like the feeling of trying something new, and I got very good at picking myself up to start again when things didn't go as planned.

Steve braced himself every time he heard the words, "I have an absolutely brilliant idea!" and was quick to ask, "How much is this one going to cost?" But when I needed a lawyer's mind or a contact or someone to brainstorm with, he was my secret weapon.

I ventured into the clothing business after seeing so many patients come to me with urinary tract and vaginal infections that were clearly caused by their thong underwear, which was wicking bacteria that belonged in the digestive tract toward the urinary and reproductive tracts, where they could cause a lot of trouble. It seemed like a simple enough problem to solve—stop wearing thongs!—but that wasn't going to happen. Many of my patients were actresses and high-profile professionals for whom visible panty lines were more than a punch line. These women were so keen to avoid ripples and ridges in their sleek clothing that they'd rather deal with infections than put on safer underwear.

So, with a good understanding of women's bodies—but not a whit of experience in design—I decided to develop a better thong. I sketched out my idea on paper. The narrow part of the garment was the troublemaker, so it needed to be wider. Any elastic had to lie flat. And this new, improved panty had to be as invisible as what it was replacing.

I bought packages of inexpensive Hanes underwear that had a shape roughly similar to what I was after, cutting and trying on versions until I had a template. It had fabric triangles that were the same size front and back, connected by a cotton crotch. The whole thing had a butterfly shape when you laid it flat, so I called it the butterfly panty.

I was stymied about how to turn my basic design into something my patients could wear until a friend mentioned a lingerie shop owner who generally just sold retail items but also made items for special clients as a gift. I showed the man my design, and, though it wasn't in his usual vocabulary, he agreed to make some samples for me.

It was an expensive way to go, and the cost limited me to ordering just five hundred pairs, but I was proud and pleased to be able to offer my butterfly panty to style-conscious women who'd now be protecting their health, too.

Steve wasn't keen on having a house full of butterfly panties on top of all those pink period kits, so I contacted a PR person I knew to get the word out. We got lucky. One small mention in *Shape* magazine at holiday time had us scrambling to fill orders. Stunned to have actual customers, I rushed to buy cute packaging material, and in the weeks before Christmas, Steve, Daniel, and I turned the kitchen table into shipping central, wrapping, packing, and sending out every last pair. In the most unexpected of Christmas miracles, we sold out.

The next "absolutely brilliant" idea was a long-simmering dream, and a much bigger production. Back when I was a resident at County, I'd begun to fantasize about how great it would be if we could get women to take better care of themselves. Most of our patients waited to come in until they were alarmed by their symptoms, and often, simple problems were crises by the time we saw them.

I wanted to make the idea of seeing a doctor less onerous. In the scenario that my mind drifted to over many years, I'd be able to offer not just checkups and procedures, but the sorts of information and treatments that could make a huge difference in women's health. There would be nutrition consultations and massage, even beauty treatments. "Alone time" and massage aren't an extravagance if your body responds negatively to stress, as so many of ours do. They're health-giving actions that can keep blood pressure and stress hormones in a manageable zone—as well as provide one of nature's great healers: pleasure. Looking good, too, is excellent for health and overall well-being. If I could create something that was a cross between a medical office and a spa, I thought, women might begin to see my offices as a place where they could come to focus on themselves and their health, not just put out fires or wait for bad news. In such an atmosphere, I thought, they'd be more likely to come for follow-up exams and to fill prescriptions. We'd hear about and address concerns early. Small problems would stay small.

The idea percolated in the background until I drove past a Victorian house in Santa Monica, just a block from the palisades park that overlooks the ocean. Perhaps I'd seen it before, but on this day, about a year into my solo practice, the house caught my attention because of the "for rent" sign out front. I knew instantly that this was the spot for my spa and "health oasis." The opposite of a cold medical office, it felt like an airy, light-filled home, and I knew we could make it warm and welcoming.

This particular *I Love Lucy* impulse was a big step. I'd have to move my offices, decorate, explain the concept to patients old and new, and, most important, assemble and pay a nurturing, talented staff. Bit by bit, it all came together. Steve swallowed hard and wrote extra checks so I could hire a top-notch physical therapist, a woman I'd referred patients to when I was in Dr. Jackson's office. She offered massage and pregnancy massage, as well as physical therapy, when that was called for. We found a nutritionist and an acupuncturist who could help patients get back in balance or even elicit contractions in a woman who was overdue to deliver. An aesthetician did facials and waxing, and our yoga teacher not only did prenatal and "mommy and me" yoga, but also labor and delivery classes. Perfect for our practice, she was also a doula.

The synergy among us was powerful. And for the couple of years we pulled together—the staff began to scatter into other businesses after that—we saw our hard work pay off in all the ways I'd hoped. We became a place where women felt supported, not rushed. Not a forbidding doctor's office, but an oasis devoted to health.

The pressure of keeping all my plates spinning made me long for a vacation. Once the spa was up and running, I started planning a trip to Paris. All those years of studying French and I'd still never been to Europe. It was the long-nourished fantasy of the girl who'd played French bingo in first grade and pasted photos of the Left Bank into her middle-school collages. I wanted everything to be perfect. We'd spend half the trip in Saint-Tropez, then ride first class to Paris on a high-speed train. There, we'd stay in a top-floor suite overlooking the Eiffel Tower and the Louvre.

Saint-Tropez was beautiful, and I pinched myself to be sure that I was walking the French Riviera with Daniel and Steve. My French was just beginning to come back to me—it had been supplanted at County by Spanish, and I still got my languages confused—when I got a frantic call from my office. "It's *Oprah*," my receptionist said. "The show. Call them right back—you can't miss this."

I was mystified. I didn't have a book or movie to sell, and as far as I knew she wasn't familiar with my work. But when I called back, a producer explained that they wanted to reprise a popular segment I'd done on *What Should You Do?* If I could make it back to Chicago in time for the taping, my team from the show would retell the story of a pregnant woman who'd fallen from a landing and been stuck through the chest with the pole of a microphone stand. I'd be the medical expert who explained the basic first-aid principle: If you're ever impaled on something, don't remove the impaling object. And I'd answer any questions that came up about what might happen to the baby in such a situation.

"I'm in France right now, and I'd have to work out a lot of logistics," I told the producer. "I'll call you back."

"You didn't just tell *Oprah* you'd call them back, did you?" Steve said, getting agitated. "That's a once in a lifetime thing, honey. If you need to go, let's just call it a vacation and go back to the States."

"But this trip is once in a lifetime, too," I replied. "I've waited for this since I was little."

"Don't be silly," he said. "We'll come back. When do they want you to be there?"

We had to take a sleeper train to get to my Chicago-bound plane in Paris, and we found ourselves crammed into a space with three narrow bunks and three or four other people in the compartment. It was cold and rainy, and excited as I was to be meeting Oprah, I was near tears at seeing my lovingly planned vacation unravel. Daniel saw how upset I was. "Mom," he said with a big smile, "sometimes things that are fun aren't always nice. I'm having fun."

It was one of the most philosophical statements I'd ever heard, especially from a fourteen year old. A cramped night train to Paris in the rain could be fun? Actually, I realized, it was. The trip to Chicago would be fun, too.

Even so, it pained me to leave Steve and Daniel in our gorgeous hotel. I'd go do the program, then fly back for one last day and night—and the boys promised they wouldn't enjoy themselves too much without me.

I was beyond jet lagged when I got to Chicago, but the producers picked me up and took me to the set so I'd be familiar with it, and perhaps be less nervous at the taping the next day. As I was standing with them, trying to keep my eyes open, Oprah glided down a grand staircase and came over to say hello. I was completely starstruck. I'd heard people talk about her presence, a sort of aura that she had, but I'd never picked it up watching her on TV. In person, though, she had a powerful charisma. I shook her hand and hoped I didn't look as terrible as I felt.

Apparently, I had. "You clean up pretty good," she said when she saw me the next day. She smiled when I explained I'd just come in from Paris ("I love that city," she said), and when our segment came up, she was full of questions for me about delivering babies ("Do they deliver themselves?").

I can't say that I was rested, or even less stressed, when we got home. But no question about it—I'd had a lot of fun.

Twenty-six

Daniel's Mom

Daniel has always been my great teacher. From the day he smiled up at me from the baby carrier on my chest and made me fall in love with him, he's been my guide. He's always had the uncanny ability to help me adjust my perspective, just as he did on that rainy train ride from Paris, and looking through his eyes, I've sometimes discovered the better version of myself and our family.

It was hard for me at first to wrap my mind around sharing my baby with Steve. That sounds odd, but I hadn't had a father in my day-to-day life, and I had to learn not to feel jealous when Daniel was out in the stroller with Steve or resting in his arms. "This kid gets a mom and a dad, and that's a good thing," I had to keep telling myself. "It's okay for him to have time alone with Steve. It's okay if they bond."

I struggled mightily with my "He's your baby, too" issues in those early months when I was a full-time mom. Daniel was all I wanted. But a different sort of reality set in when I went back to school and plunged into life at County. I thank my lucky stars that my boy is resilient. He survived when the people he saw the most were day-care workers and none of us noticed his teeth were rotting, and he thrived when Joanne, who'd moved in to care for Mom, stayed to look after him.

Through those wildly busy years when Steve and I were establishing ourselves in our new professions, I had the fantasy that if we just worked hard enough, we could give our boy the kind of security I didn't have as a kid. My mom and I had to stand together against the world—all those landlords and bill collectors—and I didn't want Daniel ever to have worries about money. I had been so responsible as a kid that even when I played I was on a mission to prove I deserved what my mom had given me, because I knew how easily it could all be taken away. I wanted Daniel simply to be a little boy. And I wanted to give him the kind of home that wasn't built clumsily from yellow lined paper. I imagined that we'd steep him in carefree luxury—the sort of "all inclusive" life I'd seen when I visited my childhood classmates. But the reality was that a leap like that wasn't going to happen in one generation.

What I could do, I realized over time, was share my many enthusiasms—and my life—with my son. My mom was precious to me because I knew her humanity, good, bad, and ugly. She was my hero, but I knew her as a real person, perfect in her imperfection. I wanted Daniel to know me that way—what I think, what I do, what I like. I wanted to be real with him. I hadn't come from Steve's *Leave It to Beaver* world, and while I could romanticize it, it's not what I was aiming for with my son. Unless maybe my June Cleaver could be more like Lucille Ball.

I love animals, so there were pets. We got Daniel a rabbit when he was a year and a half old, a sweet ball of fur that we kept until I dreamed that it was a demon rabbit with fang teeth and couldn't quite trust it anymore. Then came a ring-necked parakeet that we loved but turned out to be allergic to, a lizard, a tortoise, a saltwater tank of delicate yellow and orange seahorses (those were definitely for me), and finally, a sweet cocker spaniel puppy that took to Daniel when we stopped in a pet store just before his seventh birthday.

Steve was against getting a dog, but this puppy clearly loved our little boy, licking his hand and cuddling against him. I couldn't get that dog out of my head, so the day after we left the store empty-handed, I ran back to get it. "Just keep him here," I told the clerk. "I haven't quite worked out the arrangements yet."

That night, in classic Lucy fashion, I made Steve and Daniel's favorite dinner (that alone was enough to arouse suspicion, coming from a professed noncook), smiled a lot, and worked up to mentioning the puppy.

"Honey, you know that dog we saw yesterday?"

"Right, the one we didn't get because we're not getting a dog," Steve said.

"Um, honey . . ."

"Oh, no."

"I got the dog."

Daniel was so excited that it was impossible to renege, and the pup—we called him Lucky—joined the family. He and Daniel grew up together.

The year Daniel turned eight, we were still living in the big house we'd rented to accommodate Christopher and Mom as she was dying. Joanne was still with us, but when our landlord suddenly decided to move back into the house, we began to rethink our own life. Joanne came with us to the new place, but within a year, we decided we were ready to go on as a family without her.

That was a shock. Suddenly, there was transportation to work out, and after-school care, the logistics of a life that was complicated by my unpredictable schedule and Steve's out-of-town travel. Those were the years of truly sharing my world with Daniel. Babies arrive on their own timetables, as do emergency surgeries, and when I had to run to the hospital after picking him up, or in the middle of the night, Daniel often came with me. "Which hospital?"

he'd say as we got in the car. Before long he knew which cafeterias had the best food and what to order in each one. He also knew the door codes to all the doctors' lounges, where he'd sit and do homework or watch TV as he waited for me.

One of our more memorable times together was the night I had to get him up after midnight so I could deliver a baby. As I settled him into the lounge to wait, I reminded him, as I always did, not to put his feet on the seats. When I went to fetch him at three a.m., there he was, sitting completely upright as he slept. I felt terrible, but we turned the night into an adventure, putting down the top of the car and singing at the top of our lungs. He was Robin to my Batman.

I had to remind myself often that Daniel wasn't me. After a big fight with Steve when Daniel was in grade school, I ran into my son's room and ranted against his father but stopped short when I realized that Daniel wasn't going to rush to my defense. "Why doesn't he side with me," I puzzled. It was the reasoning of a girl who'd decided to pledge allegiance to her mom, and reject her father, at age three. And Daniel was not that child. He had two parents he loved equally, and I realized that despite my possessiveness, I'd been successful in helping guide him to that place. I knew rationally that it was a good thing. And in the face of my son's steady love for both of us, eventually, I could feel the grace of it replacing the stubborn wish that he'd love me more.

It went without saying that Daniel would go to the sorts of rigorous private schools I'd attended, but there, too, I had to let my son handle his life his own way. I was knocked back on my heels when he didn't do an extra-credit section of a test in middle school and go for the A-plus over an A.

"You had a chance for extra credit and you didn't take it?" I said. "Why not?"

"Because I already did well," he answered.

"But you could've done better," I insisted.

After enough exchanges like that, it occurred to me that not everyone needs the A-plus-plus. And it was quite all right if my laid-back boy didn't feel driven in the same way I had. I didn't have to push him so hard. He wasn't me. That was a hard concept for me—and I think it's a hard one for lots of parents. But Daniel stayed true to himself, and finally, I got it. I'm the one who always somehow wants to make myself better. He's the one who's confident and at ease with himself. Yes, he has my smile, he moves like me, and we like the same music—but he's his own person.

We bonded over his school sports. I sat in the bleachers as he and his tiny-tyke soccer team wandered around the field, distracted by butterflies and uninterested in the ball. Later, it was baseball, then swimming and wrestling. As a mom, you feel everything, whether it's a twisted ankle or a hard fall or the disappointment of a loss. Those things and the tedium of driving. And waiting. I did try to multitask. My son heard me on the phone with patients so much in the car that when he was quite young he asked, "How come women have so many yeast infections?" He probably knew the standard advice for any number of women's ob/gyn concerns.

Into the six-ring circus of our lives, I'd occasionally drop a sports fixation of my own and send us on a wild chase for lessons and equipment. I'd wanted to surf since Bishop's, where I'd always had secret crushes on the rangy surfer boys, and when Daniel was six or seven, I heard about a La Jolla group called the Surf Divas that taught women to handle a board. On my days off, I'd load up

Joanne and Daniel and head down for a lesson. Daniel tried it once, but he was still too small to enjoy it yet, so those were beach days for him. I'd surf an hour or two, and we'd drive home with the top down on the Mustang, stopping for burritos. On a family trip to Hawaii a couple of years later, we all took lessons, and this time Daniel was able to stand up on the board. We came home promising ourselves we'd do more.

The opportunity presented itself almost immediately. In a surf shop where we'd gone to buy a skateboard, we were approached by a man with a South African accent who asked if we surfed. He introduced himself as a teacher, gave us his number, and in short order Daniel was taking regular lessons after school, working his way up from a beginner's board to a short board. We were close enough to his teacher that he was the one I turned to when I was caught in surgery late one afternoon. I called him on a speakerphone, told him I was in the OR, and asked him to pick up Daniel and take him out to the water.

During those years all of us went out with our boards every weekend. I had just set up my new office and spa, and some weeks were crazily busy with work and media obligations, but in the waves with Daniel on my pink surfboard, all of that washed away.

Other sports phases came and went. In-line skating on Venice Beach. Fly-fishing. Horseback riding. That last was another item from my "always wanted to try it" list. I'd mooned over the equestrian program when I was at Mount Holyoke, longing to ride with the team but cowed by the expense of it. And of course, I knew nothing about dressage. At the time it was one of those easy choices: Do you want to be a doctor, or would you rather hang out with horses? But once I was out of school, I thought I might be able to do both.

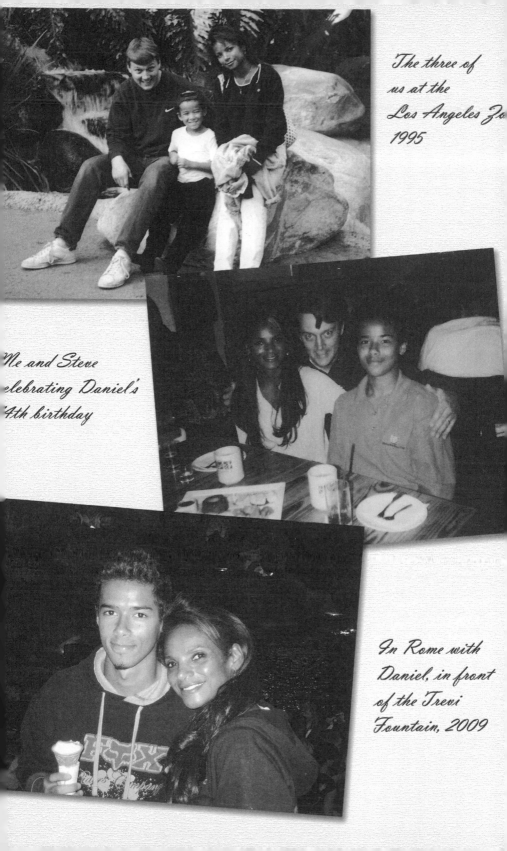

The three of
us at the
Los Angeles Zo
1995

Me and Steve
celebrating Daniel's
4th birthday

In Rome with
Daniel, in front
of the Trevi
Fountain, 2009

Daniel was game to try riding with me, and we took a few family vacations at dude ranches, where I could climb onto a gentle mare and he could ride a pony. We found a club in Malibu where we could ride and play tennis and took a few lessons up there, too, but riding went the way of skating.

As for the fly-fishing, it was a moment. Like a lot of women, I suspect, I was romanced by the idea of it when I saw *A River Runs Through It*, the '90s Brad Pitt movie based on the Norman Maclean story. The vision that lingered in my head years later was powerful enough to override my childhood fishing trauma—the hook in the hand with Grandpa—and send me to the bookstore to read up on the lore. I got a kit for making lures, remembering how one of my Nutella friends from college had made bracelets fashioned from them—and we loaded up on long bamboo fishing rods and maps of nearby lakes. When a summer's worth of attempts didn't yield a single fish, I put aside the fantasy and moved on. Steve always tried everything, knowing that the jag would probably pass soon enough.

Through it all, Daniel persevered with karate, an activity that belonged solely to him, practicing and competing all the way through high school. I was there as he advanced to black belt and there to pick him up the day he took a mighty leap and landed with a sickening force with his legs splayed in the splits. I knew he was hurt and instantly phoned a friend in the ER. It was an excruciating injury—he'd torn his hamstring off the hipbone and spent the next weeks on crutches.

It was an accident I'd have given anything to avoid, but we grew close in those halting days of recovery, as we did after another childhood injury, when he was using a new Swiss Army knife to dislodge a marble from the neck of a Japanese soda bottle. The knife flipped, and he came out of his room saying, "I think I cut myself." I took him into the bathroom to rinse the cut and figure out how deep it was, and I could see that it was down to the bone. He went pale and began to crumple, and I tried to catch him, but we both wound up on the floor.

I gathered him up, wrapped his hand, and rushed him to the emergency room, where an orthopedist I'd called stitched him back together. It was a frantic day made even more so because I was to interview for an on-camera slot at CNN that afternoon. Daniel and I were both dazed, but once his finger was sewn together and in a splint, and we'd made an appointment for him to see a hand specialist the next day, there was nothing to do but keep going. We drove from the hospital to the studio, and I took him along to the interview, where the consensus was that I looked "too young" for the job, though I felt as if I'd just aged a hundred years.

The knife had cut cleanly through a tendon, and Daniel would need surgery to reattach it, as well as long weeks of physical therapy to regain the full use of his finger. In a practical sense that meant we were joined at the hip—he had to go to the office with me so we could make the therapy appointment after work. It was a long, long summer for him. But on days I could finish early, we'd go for a sushi and talk—a small treat to look forward to. And over the weeks it became our tradition, talking over lunch, reconnecting

We still do that, and it's gotten us through the times when it's been a strain having a crazy surfing mom with strange pets, TV gigs, pregnant patients, and a panty business.

Just as Mom wasn't the most traditional mother around, I admit that I've been outside the box myself. But like her I think I've given my child a real sense of who I am, and I've appreciated as much of him as I can. The man who grew from that baby with the intense, insistent gaze is a calm, beautiful soul who can flow with whatever the world throws at him. And it's a good thing, too—because at our house you never know what's coming next.

Twenty-seven

Opportunity

The husband of one of my patients was an Olympic runner from Ghana, whom I got to know over the many months of prenatal visits. "Have you ever been to my country?" he asked early on.

"No," I said, "the closest I've been is the Philippines, and that's not too close."

It was a routine exchange, on par with "Nice weather," but as we continued to talk, and I described the charity work we'd done in the Philippines, he began tell me about the need for medical services in his country. "Maybe you would think of coming," he said after one of our visits. "I can connect you with the minister of health."

Almost spontaneously, we began to hatch a plan. The Ghanaian health minister contacted me and said he'd heard I was considering an aid trip. If I gave him a date, he said, he'd put me in touch with a hospital and arrange for me to help out with surgeries and deliveries in the obstetrics ward.

I looked up Ghana on the Internet. It's a small country (about the size of Indiana and Illinois combined) in West Africa, the segment of the continent that bulges into the Atlantic before the land mass tapers toward the Cape of Good Hope. Ghana sits on the bottom of that bulge, between Ivory Coast and Togo, bordering the Gulf of Guinea. It's a stable democracy, the world's second largest producer of cocoa. And its infant mortality rate, about sixty-four deaths per one thousand births, was reasonably good for sub-Saharan Africa. (In the United States, which ranked thirtieth in the world, about seven infants died per thousand births.) But my patient's husband, after hearing my descriptions of what we'd encountered in the Philippines, said I should probably be braced for similar conditions.

I had long meant to return to humanitarian work, and now, with my practice on its feet, this invitation had appeared. The timing seemed right, not just for a trip but for starting my own charity. Opportunities hadn't come easily in my life. They were seized, begged for, and conjured, sometimes, out of little more than fast talking and desire. But I've worked hard to share their fruit. I'll probably spend the rest of my life making sure that the gifts that have found their way into my hands will not be squandered. I can't give back what my mother took for me, but I can pour my talents into the world. Maybe it's the beginning of a repayment.

In 2005, the year we decided to start the charity, we didn't really have the money to fund it. Steve and I were still working toward the plus side of the ledger. But I could donate my services, Steve could donate his for the paperwork involved in setting up a 501-C3 nonprofit, and somehow, we thought, we'd come up with the resources we needed for a Ghana trip and, perhaps, others.

My time in the Philippines had given me a basic sense of the supplies that we'd probably want to take, and my office staff and I took every opportunity to ask local hospitals if they had extra suture sets and surgical supplies they'd be willing to donate. We chatted up drug reps to see if their companies would make donations of money or medicine. And we made friends at the Red Cross in Santa Monica, which let us have stickers for our bags that would, we hoped, identify them as relief supplies instead of contraband. Our medical staff for the initial Ghana trip would consist of me and one of the nurses from the office, and Daniel and Steve would come along to give us whatever support we needed once we arrived.

This was our first global seat-of-the-pants effort, and we paid for our lack of savvy. For all our preparations, we didn't realize we needed visas to enter Ghana, and we were detained in a dank room at the airport for hours as officials there searched our bags and threatened to send us home. Finally, Steve stumbled on the magic words: How much for a visa? And in exchange for an amount of cash he's never revealed ("It wasn't as bad as I thought it might be," is all he's ever told me), the immigration officials sent us on our way with the documents we needed.

We checked into a small hotel run by a Chinese couple and got our bearings. It was hot, almost dizzyingly so, and the hospital offered no reprieve. I had taken for granted the air-conditioning in the simple but modern operating room Dr. Lagasse had built in the Philippines, but here I learned why it had been so important. I'd be doing C-sections and other procedures for the next seven days in a large cement room equipped with a wrought iron operating table topped by a thin pad. Without air-conditioning, the smells of blood and bodily fluids, usually neutralized by cool air, were overpowering. Flies flew in the open windows and landed on the bodies I was working on, and the nurse would shoo them away.

With no residents or trained physicians to assist me, I literally didn't have enough hands to do surgery, so on the first day I pulled Daniel into the OR and showed him how to retract the flesh around incisions for me. I'd seen many a med student faint at the sight of blood in surgery, and the smells here only added to the sensory assault. But if he was squeamish, he didn't let on, though he was only fourteen then, and I'm sure being thrown into surgery that way left a deep impression. I thought back to my first view of the OR when I was his age and remembered how enthralled I'd been. I quietly hoped he'd have at least a touch of that fascination.

Like the patients I'd seen at County, most of the women I'd been scheduled to treat had had scant prenatal care, and I was there to help those survivors survive. We'd missed the easy interventions like nutritional supplements, medicines, rest, and screenings to determine if the fetus was developing normally. Now there were often complications to deal with. It was common to see patients whose high blood pressure or diabetes had gone untreated for the length of their pregnancies and who could easily have died without a crash C-section. Hemorrhages were often fatal here. Infections were a constant threat because sanitation in the hospital couldn't approach the standards in the wards where I'd worked and trained. It was factors like these that drove infant mortality rates to a level nine times higher than those in the United States.

At County the onslaught of high-risk women was overwhelming, but there, equipment was modern and working and patients had access to highly skilled specialists. Here, a woman's chances were as good as the doctor treating her, and deliveries, no matter how complicated, could be in the hands of physicians who had only a glancing knowledge of obstetrics. Fetal monitors, those simple, vital tools for keeping tabs on the distress of a baby during labor, were few—I had one only because I brought it with me. And other equipment was old, sometimes failing.

Every once in a while, a patient's stats would plummet on the monitors, and I learned to ask the anesthesiologist to check the oxygen mask. It had been duct-taped together, and when the tape worked loose, oxygen would flow into the room instead of into the patient's lungs. A quick adjustment was generally all it took to bring us back from the brink—but the patient had been needlessly endangered. In the midst of complicated surgeries, we were forced to improvise, and the process was bumpy. But it worked. Women lived through hemorrhages. Babies squalled into the world after emergency C-sections. And at the end of a long day of surgery,

Daniel and I would walk back to the hotel, exhausted but satisfied. The needs were tremendous, but we were facing them, one mother at a time.

Steve had been excited about the possibilities of the charity, which we'd decided to call Maternal Fetal Care International, or MFCI. He'd always wanted to travel, and we both envisioned him as having a sort of CEO role. On this first trip he brought a video camera and interviewed the hospital staff, documenting our work and trying to find out what was needed. His reconnaissance work, I thought, could enhance our ability to make a difference wherever we decided to go.

But the heat, and the stress of being in the midst of such a voracious demand for our aid, with such limited means to help, set us on edge.

"I'm beginning to wonder why I'm here," Steve said wearily.

"All those babies and moms," I replied. "That's why we're here."

"But I'm not so sure about me," he complained. "You're the doctor, you're the one they need. I don't know what I'm doing here."

Tangling with African officials, eating greasy Chinese food for every meal, day after day—I knew it was wearing on all of us. Daniel longed for a hamburger, and our homesick nurse longed to leave. I think the worst part of the trip for Steve was that on some level it made him think again about how different he is from me. I was a proven "jump in, try to do some good, and don't worry about perfection" type—and I had gotten a lot of projects off the ground because of it. Not all of them would fly, and I'd realize sometimes that I didn't want to keep them up and running. But I tried, learned from my mistakes, tried again. We were saving lives in Africa because of it.

Steve had a lawyer's mind and an innate sense of wanting everything to be just right before he'd put his name on it. He'd made partner at his firm because of that devotion to detail and polish. But it got in his way sometimes. He was a talented writer, and he wanted to have finished a book by now, but perfectionist that he was, he couldn't bring himself to bang out a bad first draft that he could shine to a high gloss. He could only see the "bad" in an effort like that, not the possibilities. And when he saw me having fun dreaming up underwear or putting together a trip to Africa, I think it felt as though I were taunting him. It seemed to me that he couldn't see how much he'd contributed in his own way—how much time and how many ideas and resources he'd come up with to help those projects gel. We were a team, and a powerful one, but he couldn't feel it. Maybe I didn't remind him often enough. The trip to Ghana was the last relief mission he took with me. Daniel wouldn't join me again, either. What he saw left him somewhat shaken. Yet I'm so glad they went, and I'm glad for the lives they helped save. I know they are, too.

I don't think I considered when I set out for Ghana that I might be taking a risk. As we were leaving, the chief of the hospital came by to thank me. "We're so happy that you did all these operations and no one has died," he said. The truth was, women and babies often died in the middle of procedures like the ones I'd performed. Often, the surgeon was an internist whose training consisted of one appendectomy and one C-section, a doctor whose only measure of whether he'd done subsequent operations correctly was if the patient lived. Care was frequently rationed on the basis of who had the $50 to pay for anesthesia or the $11 to cover the price of the sutures for their surgery. Patients would be sent to the market to buy their own stitches, and if the fee were too princely, they might die of a simple condition or bleed to death. Death was a common outcome. Yet I wondered what might've happened if I'd lost one of my patients, all that despair and anger aimed at stranger. I couldn't dwell on things that hadn't happened, though. Our trip had been a success. We were going home.

Now there was a charity to fund, and it was time to learn how. There was so much need—but it was fixable if we could round up the resources. At first we failed miserably. I sent solicitations to patients and friends, but there are lots of people asking for money, and my requests seemed to fall into a black hole. I rejiggered the strategy for attempt number two, teaming up with a maker of maternity clothes to put on a fashion show in my office. That raised enough for more plane tickets and supplies. My next fund-raiser would be more ambitious. I just wasn't sure what shape it would take.

Toward the end of that year I got a call from Dr. Lagasse. I hadn't spoken to him for months, if not years, but he'd thought of me when UCLA was looking for someone to oversee gynecology residents in a program it was operating in Eritrea. I jumped at the chance to go back to Africa and extend the reach of MFCI—even if MFCI was still essentially just me.

I filled in for a doctor who'd been scheduled to handle gynecology surgeries and met the residents. Eritrea was politically unsettled—and concerns about the safety of the medical residents ultimately led UCLA to dissolve their program. But I felt strangely at home there. People often mistook me for Eritrean, and in their confusion there was a comforting embrace.

Near the end of the trip, my office called with an urgent message. It was a producer from *Oprah*—it seems I have to be very far away to register on their radar—inviting me to make a solo appearance on the show. I had to laugh. It was one thing to get from Paris

*Alfre Woodard, Marianne Jean-Baptiste, me,
and Cookie Johnson at the MFCI fundraiser,
May 8, 2007 Photo credit: Ray Mickshaw*

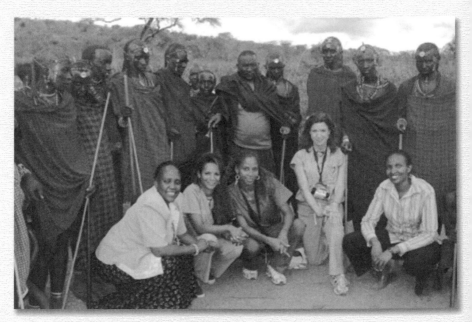

*Me, Holly Robinson Peete, and Donna Lane in our scrubs
in Africa for MFCI (2007)*

to Chicago. Getting there from Eritrea was more complicated. I hated to miss the opportunity, but I knew it would probably vanish when I laid out what it would take: They'd need to fly me in from Africa, then fly me home, as returning to Asmara (Eritrea's capital city) would be pointless. If I left early, someone else would have taken over my surgeries.

I was startled when the producer got back to me to say the arrangements had been made. I'd be on a show for a long segment; I'd be answering questions about women's health. This time I'd be on stage alone with Oprah. It seems they'd remembered me from that first appearance and had been keeping up with my work since.

The show was a popular one—those common questions about fibroids and sexuality and heavy periods always find an interested audience—and when I had a chance to tell Oprah about my charity and the work in Africa, I felt as though my worlds were coming together. Mom always said, "Shoot higher; what else can we do?" Now I had the chance, at least once, to reach a huge audience of women with positive messages about their health. And maybe in time there would be opportunities as well to reach people with a vision of what we could do for women and babies in places like Ghana and Eritrea given equipment and education and $11 packages of sutures.

TWENTY-EIGHT

Charity

The world seemed to open up once we launched the charity. Dr. Lagasse's group, "Medicine for Humanity," was returning to the Philippines in February of 2006, and I was invited to join them, taking MFCI to provide ob/gyn surgery and supplies. Separately, a doctor I knew in India invited me to come there. I thought I might make both stops on one trip.

As those seeds were germinating, and I was planning for my travels, I was asked to do a commercial for a fertility watch, an intriguing device that picks up the changes in a woman's salt ions and lets her know when she's ovulating. While we filmed, I chatted about MFCI with the person behind the camera, a woman named Donna Lane, and on the spot she offered to join me in India, where she'd document the work I'd be doing there.

Steve wasn't wild about my timing. We were in the throes of planning our largest fund-raiser yet, an event we called the Lullaby Ball. This time I'd reached into my community of patients and media contacts to find celebrities to support MFCI. Poppy Montgomery and Marianne Jean-Baptiste of the TV drama *Without a Trace*; Tava Smiley, the TV host and reporter; and Alfre Woodard of *Desperate Housewives* were among the bold-face names we attracted this time, and we'd seen an enthusiastic response to an auction that offered as its grand prize a trip with me on one of my relief missions.

It would've been smart to stay home to handle the complicated logistics, but I didn't want to miss a chance to cement relationships with hospitals and doctors in places MFCI could do good work. So I made the trip, delivering supplies and plunging into rounds of surgery in overstressed, underequipped settings. These travels were part bonding, part scouting, part sightseeing, and I was glad for Donna's company in India, where she filmed one of the C-sections I performed and documented the labor room, where two women shared a bed. Once more I was seeing patients who were being denied lifesaving procedures because they didn't have even the small amount of money that would pay for sutures, and much of my time was spent trying to undo the effects of avoidable complications.

Donna and I let off steam by trying to take in our surroundings—visiting temples, buying saris and bangles, letting local children advise us on what to eat. We took more footage at a village where many of the children had lost their mothers at birth. It was sensory and emotional overload, but it made even our limited efforts seem worthwhile. The United Nations had set a number of millennium development goals, aiming to improve conditions around the world between 1990 and 2015, and two in particular spoke loudly to me. The first was to reduce by two-thirds the mortality rate of infants and children under age five. The second was to reduce the maternal mortality rate by two-thirds. MFCI was small, but we could put our resources, as they grew, behind that effort.

The Lullaby Ball, with its red-carpet turnout, raised $70,000, a huge sum for us, though it was a pittance compared with the millions that well-established fund-raisers bring in in Los Angeles. We'd use every dollar to take services back to Africa and Asia. In the fall Dr. Lagasse's group invited me to join them in Kenya, and I decided to go with Marianne Jean-Baptiste, who wanted to learn more about MFCI.

The trip went badly. The hospital where I had planned to offer my services didn't seem to need them, and I had the sinking feeling that our time and expenses had been donated for naught. There was tension, too—I think the presence of a celebrity made for confusion among the other visiting doctors, who seemed to keep us at arm's length. Discouraged, we decided to split from the group and find a place where we could do some good.

A woman at the hospital had relatives at a Maasai village in a southern area called Ngatatek, and she not only urged us to visit but came with us to the village hospital. She was also able to arrange a meeting with the minister of health, who described the needs of the area. Here, transportation and geography were key factors in the life and death of women and infants. Women often had to walk forty or fifty miles to reach a hospital where they could receive prenatal care or give birth, and a clean, centrally located clinic could cut travel time—and risks of death—significantly.

We were on our own in a country we didn't know, but we thought we could help. The health minister and the village elders— a stately group in vivid traditional dress—agreed to let us have a one-room clinic for a "birthing shack" if we would equip it as a delivery room and teach the area doctor and nurse, as well as the elderly women who often attended births, how to provide prenatal care.

I returned twice that year, the first time to set up the new clinic and establish prenatal protocols and the second to deliver the clinic's first baby. I tracked down a used but functional delivery table and a bed where women could rest before and after giving birth. I think the businessman I dealt with looked at me as an easy mark and ratcheted up his prices, but I'm a good bargainer and managed to bring them back down to earth. The equipment arrived to great excitement in the community—so much so that the pieces were assembled right out on the dirt in front of our clinic and had to be broken down once more when they wouldn't fit through the door.

Our priority on that first trip back was to teach the staff what to do on each prenatal visit, basic procedures that could catch problems early. We brought blood pressure cuffs and showed the nurse and doctor how to use them, along with scales for weighing the patients, urine cups, and a notebook for keeping track of each woman. The centerpiece of the teaching effort was a chart we taped to the wall that spelled out the steps of a checkup: (1) take blood pressure; if it's above this level or below this level, send the patient to the district hospital; (2) measure weight; if the patient has gained this much over the standard, send her to the district hospital. There were similar directives for urine dips and fundal height measurements—tracking the size of the "baby bump"—procedures that we wanted to institute as part of a routine visit. It's simple stuff, mundane even, but putting basic monitoring in place means that a woman who has a condition like preeclampsia, as I did with Daniel, will be able to get help navigating the dangers of her high blood pressure and, with luck, have a safe delivery.

Few of my patients at home could imagine going through their pregnancies without regular visits to check their vital signs, peek in on the growing baby with ultrasounds, and monitor eating habits or conditions such as anemia. Harder still is imagining visits that might require a walk of ten miles, twenty miles, or more on swollen feet that might be barely visible below an expanding belly. To make such a walk while in labor is almost unfathomable, yet that's what might be required if a Maasai mother wanted her baby to be delivered in the simplest of modern clinics. It's extremely difficult to calculate the hazards to mothers under such circumstances, though a 2005 estimate put the lifetime risk of dying in childbirth in Kenya at one in thirty-nine. With limited access to modern medical technology, and hazardous customs such as restricting the diet of expectant moms (so babies will be smaller and, it's reasoned, easier to deliver), it's likely that the risks for Maasai women are even greater.

Reaching the Ngatatek village isn't easy. It's a two-hour drive from Nairobi via washboard roads, and the hazards are many. The U.S. State Department has been warning for years of potential dangers to travelers. The country has seen bombings, kidnappings, beheadings, and mayhem, threats we put out of our minds until we were stopped at a border by armed men. I didn't tell my husband about incidents like that or mention our close encounters with the hippos that we belatedly noticed within charging distance when we stopped for a break. We were, after all, traveling through wild, stunning plains studded with stark acacia trees and wildlife. It was hard to take it all in. Mostly, we hung on for dear life as we bounced in our truck clutching our supplies.

The Maasai appeared, seemingly from thin air, each time we came, gathering in front of the clinic. On our second trip a woman we'd met earlier was ready to deliver, and her family, the village chiefs, and a group of elderly women came to wait with her. On this trip I was joined by Holly Robinson Peete, an actress I'd been watching since *Hangin' with Mr. Cooper* in the early '90s. Holly threw on a pair of scrubs and took turns with us to walk the pregnant woman as her labor progressed. It was late evening when her water broke. One of us took cleanup duty, and I came away with a fresh appreciation for hospitals where a staff handles such tasks.

The baby—healthy and yelling—arrived around midnight, and when we went back to the local hotel where we were staying, the Maasai insisted on doing a celebratory traditional dance. Sleep would've been welcome by then, but this was a moment worth marking. We'd rest later.

I'd never traveled so much, dreamed so big, or been so humbled by the magnitude of the job in front of me. But it was thrilling to see the possibilities of this work and how substantially we could improve people's lives. Every situation I landed in was different. Here it was a birthing shed. In Eritrea it would be a vision for educating a new generation of ob/gyns.

TWENTY-NINE

Diary of a Relief Trip, Eritrea, 2007

Day One: Friday into Saturday

I've been up all night after a frantic day with two cesarean sections and one vaginal delivery, trying to see and check up on as many of my pregnant patients as I can and briefing the doctor on call for me about special and high-risk patients. I get Daniel to help me unload all the supplies from the car while I give him instructions on being safe and what he can and cannot do while I am gone. It's still tough for me to be away from him, even though he has just turned seventeen.

I'm packing the supply bag the morning of the trip because most of the Foley bags, medications, infant caps, sutures, and equipment did not arrive, of course, until the day before. I usually take two bags, one devoted to MFCI supplies and a smaller one with my clothes and scrubs, mostly scrubs.

I send Steve to the bank to make the deposits that I skipped during the week, because I haven't had a minute to go. The week before leaving on these trips is always absolute hell. I also send him to the store for my malaria medication and sundries while I shower and finish packing.

On the way to the airport, I check in with my office and on-call doctor one last time, go over Daniel's schedule with Steve, and remind him not to let our son go wild with the car or break his curfew. I know he's not a kid anymore, but it's hard to let go.

After a not-so-bad sleep from Los Angeles to Frankfurt, I do the tedious transfer routine and then go to meet my German friends and colleagues at the terminal. I'm working with a German nonprofit organization, Hammer Forum, in Eritrea, and I've taken an eight-week German course to help me communicate with these partners. I've only mastered niceties, such as "How are you" and "Nice weather," but I understand more than I used to. The German group is quite large, probably about thirty.

After stopping in Jeddah, in Saudi Arabia, we land in Asmara and step into the dark, foggy night. We walk from plane to airport under the stars and go to customs. Dr. Habteab, director of Orotta National Referral Hospital, is there to greet us and to make sure there are no problems.

Every time I've visited, something remarkable has happened: The people I meet swear that I look Eritrean and just start speaking to me in the native Tigrinya language. I usually look confused and say I'm not Eritrean. But I love it—it makes me feel welcomed and at home.

It doesn't help me at customs, though. Before I can leave, the agents have to open and inspect my bag full of supplies, which has been flagged with an "X." Dr. Habteab tries to explain that I'm just carrying medical supplies, but nonetheless they need to rummage through all the Foley catheter bags to get to the fetal Doppler. It takes me a minute to make the obvious connection: It's electronic. *That's* why it's triggered so much concern.

We leave the airport in two minibuses, and the obstetrical team winds up at the Sunshine Hotel. Our schedule for tomorrow includes a meeting with the minister of health before we go to the hospital for labor and delivery.

I settle in for the visit. My room, like much of the architecture and decor you see in Eritrea, has an Italian flavor, reflecting the country's colonial years. This hotel, like the neighboring buildings, is caught in a time warp that places it in the 1940s or '50s, and since a lot of things haven't been kept up, it's a bit like visiting your Italian grandma's rundown villa. My room smells distinctly of mothballs. There is beautiful Italian furniture, but the light fixtures are old. The tiles are peeling. So is the paint. The place is a mixture of quaint and not quite right.

Day Two: Sunday

After a restless night, I'm awakened by the call to prayer at a nearby mosque at around five a.m. The chanting fills the air as if to remind everyone to pray and meditate, whatever their religion or language (Eritrea is a largely Christian country). I open my windows and look out at Asmara—the rundown Italian villas, the people on bicycles, the palm trees and bougainvilleas. For a moment it's hard to believe I'm in Africa.

I meet the German doctors for breakfast, and we head to the hospital for the meeting with the health minister. In the conference room we are arranged by importance around a formal meeting table, with the minister of health at the head, and the president of Hammer Forum facing him.

The minister of health is a direct man. He doesn't hesitate to tell us that his most important goal is to start an obstetrics and gynecology residency program in Eritrea, and he wants us—MFCI and the Hammer Forum—to do it by January 2008, just a few months away. He stresses the importance of the timetable. The maternal mortality rate is extremely high, he reminds us, and it's rising.

Then he looks directly at me and asks me to speak. I tell him that we're excited by the important new job he has given us, but it's a huge undertaking, and January 2008 is truly unrealistic. He says that date was his goal for starting the pediatric and surgery residency he's also setting up—but maybe for our program September 2008 is more realistic. Then he goes over what the ministry will provide for the doctors who come and explains the structure of the program that he has in mind.

He wants us to design the curriculum and find a director to oversee the program from Eritrea for at least one to two years, if not more. "Wow" is my first response. The prospect is fabulous and frightening at the same time. Creating the first obstetrics and gynecology residency program in Eritrea—and perhaps creating a model for all of Africa—could be a big step toward solving the problem of maternal and infant mortality across the continent. We doctors look at each other, continue to make a few comments, and decide that we need to meet again tonight with the new medical director of the surgical residency program, since he'd have good insights to offer.

At the labor and delivery ward of the hospital, there is a long line of women who wait outside and in the hallway. The smell of blood and urine greets us at the door, along with the screaming and chanting of women in labor without pain medication. There are three women in the delivery room, and all eight beds in the labor room are full. One woman is sitting in a pool of blood after delivering in the bed. Two dead babies wrapped in green cloth lie on a table, waiting to be taken away. The midwives flurry around speaking Tigrinya as we do a quick hug-kiss meet and greet—and then go to work.

After a few deliveries, a stillbirth, and a sixteen-year-old mother who died from a postpartum hemorrhage after she arrived too late for us to save her, we return to our hotel for the meeting with the obstetrical director. I'm exhausted and hungry when I get back to my room. All I want is a Coca-Cola and a nap—but there's no time and no Coca-Cola. No Coke anywhere except in small specialty shops that import it.

We gather in the lobby, the three German doctors, the medical director, the assistant to the minister of health, and I. It feels like a landmark meeting—the beginning of something special—and one of the doctors documents everything: what I've agreed to provide for the curriculum from the United States, what the German doctors have agreed to, our time frame, our deadlines.

The biggest obstacles we can see are gaining university support and financial support for the physician stipends and providing a competent medical director to run our new program—especially since accepting the post would require taking a decreased salary and living in Eritrea for two years.

We go out for Chinese food feeling slightly overwhelmed.

Day Three: Monday

The rhythmic wake-up call from the mosque, along with some roosters in the background, rouses me for our 7:30 a.m. breakfast. I'm getting used to listening to German and trying to catch words I understand. I've tried speaking French with some of the Germans because they often understand it better than English.

Gas is scarce, so we walk to the hospital, passing women who sweep the street with palm fronds. In the traditional white head and shoulder drape, they look like black Madonnas. Everyone has delicate facial features that seem, not surprisingly, like a black and Italian blend.

We join the hospital's six Eritrean ob/gyns as they discuss the patients over traditional chai tea served in a glass tea set. When we return to labor and delivery, there are three stillbirths wrapped in green. We give the grateful matron, Miriam, the supplies that we've brought, then do two cesarean sections before a meeting at the Ministry of Health. On the agenda: a presentation on telemedicine, which is especially interesting to us now that we're thinking about the new residency program.

The meeting is cancelled, but as fortune would have it, I meet an American woman named Fatima, one of the general surgeons who have come to participate in the new general surgery residency program. That program might be a model for ours, I realize, and I pump her for details about the residency, the medical students, and how their stipend is supported. She's a bright, energetic woman—just what you'd expect from a female general surgeon from the United States—but obviously more special. When I tell her about the wonderful/daunting idea for an ob/gyn residency, she offers herself as a resource and gives me not only her cell number but also a Tigrinya phrase book, which I had been looking for everywhere. Wow!

Back at labor and delivery, a woman with a breech delivery—a rarity in the United States and Germany—is in labor. As we wait for her to progress, we show the medical students how to use ultrasound on patients, and I try to teach them about fetal heart-rate monitoring. It's my personal mission to get fetal monitoring in place, but it's going to take some work for either of these tools to be used as routinely as they are back home. The breech seemed to be doing well, and we take a break. The medical director has invited us out for an authentic Eritrean meal.

At a residence with a large gate, we wait until a woman in traditional Eritrean dress with an *nsalla*—the white wrap I'd seen draped over women's heads and shoulders—lets us in. She leads us down a long corridor in the house, where we come to a large sitting room with pictures, paintings, and knickknacks from ceiling to floor. Lining the walls are tables and chairs covered in animal skins. We sit, and *myes*, a traditional drink with honey and alcohol, is served in a beautiful glass carafe. Then comes flat bread, which one of the doctors blesses by breaking it—a ritual that feels like Communion.

Our hostess brings an ornate copper pitcher, something out of *The Arabian Nights*, filled with warm water, along with a copper bowl and soap container. In this ceremonial hand-washing, we soap and rinse our fingers under the water that she pours as if we're scrubbing for surgery. Over a dinner of meats, fish, and sauces, served buffet style, we relax and get to know each other. The director tells us he's arranged for us to go by train to see the hospital in Gindae—a great chance to see how people live outside Asmara.

Day Four: Tuesday

The train to Gindae is eighty years old, and it looks like a relic from the Old West—a front engine pulling a small passenger cabin with open windows and a trailer. The countryside flashes by, bales of hay and goats. Then I hear the train whistle blowing and sense something even more exciting going on. When I walk to the front of the passenger car and step into the open engine, followed by some of my German friends, it feels as though we're on top of the world with the wind blowing, the engineer in his cowboy hat next to me, and the smoke coming from the engine of this little toy train. We wind around the mountains of Asmara, and I look down from the heights with birds soaring around me. In the tunnels all I can feel is the rhythmic motion of the train as the world disappears into the dark, reduced to white smoke from the steam engine that curls under the curve of the roof and spreads out like a rippled blanket, casting off a magical glow chased by the "hoot, hoot" of the train.

As we pass the villages carved into the mountainsides, a strong smell of urine wafts toward us. We wave to the children who come out of the huts and shacks and see women gathering water and carrying wood along the tracks. When we pull into the first tiny station, kids crowd around the train. I ask the conductor if I can give them candy, and when I do, they gather around like pigeons in a feeding frenzy.

The final stop is a town close to Gindae, where we eat lunch and cake as women carrying wood and water lead their camels past. The conductor tells us we can't use the outhouse because someone is living in it.

A car takes us to the Gindae hospital, an empty, lovely façade— a hospital without equipment and with only one general doctor to serve an enormous area with a huge population.

We can help here, but that, too, is going to take a lot of work. The weight of the world comes back to me. But I'm cheered by a rare treat—a cold bottle of Coca-Cola. The train is sponsored by Coke.

Still covered with soot from the train ride back to Asmara, we go to check on labor and delivery. The ward is quiet, and the fetal heart-rate monitor is at least plugged in in the labor room, though no one is using it. The breech baby from the day before had been delivered vaginally, we learn, but it had lived for only thirty minutes. We go back to the hotel plunged back into despair, but there is more to do: a dinner meeting arranged by Fatima, who has pulled together the hospital's health director, the minister of health's assistant, and three people from her program—the pediatric surgeon, the general surgeon, and the director of the surgical residency program.

For once we don't need to reinvent the wheel. We talk about how our program and theirs will be similar and yet different, how we can work with the same foundation they've already built there, and how we can structure our own residency. It always feels like you are on the right track when the world or the forces out there seem to work with you. I'm in awe of the world right now. All systems seemed to be working for us to do this for the minister of health—however daunting and large the project. Start the first ob/

gyn residency program in Eritrea? Why not! The world seems to be saying yes!

Day Five: Wednesday

At the doctors' morning meeting and tea, they thank us once again for the Foley bags and for the medications we brought— some are almost impossible for them to get, they tell us. One of the doctors reports on a patient who needed an emergent cesarean hysterectomy because her uterus ruptured after a long labor with a hydrocephalic (water on the brain) baby. My OB team exchanges glances. We know that if they had performed an ultrasound on the patient, she would still have her uterus and her baby.

The infant, a boy, is wrapped in green cloth on the table when we return to the hospital. We examine the body silently, all think-ing the same thing—how unnecessary. How awful. The mother is stable but receiving her second unit of blood. We make a point of impressing on the labor and delivery director that it's necessary to do an ultrasound on every patient.

One of my last tasks on this trip is to visit a school, where I'll talk to students in hopes of helping eliminate the practice of female genital mutilation (FGM). Eritrea has one of the highest rates, at about 95 percent. In April the country passed the first law against FGM, but the custom persists. I'm to meet the German doctor, Christophe, at the Italian high school (for Eritreans) at ten-thirty.

The classroom is full, probably eighty-plus students, when we arrive. Christophe and I have agreed that it would be good to go over the past, present, and future of FGM and get their ideas about how to stop the practice. Last year we did more of an informative talk, with a great Q&A with the kids, but this year we don't have time for that. I need to get back to the hospital to examine a patient.

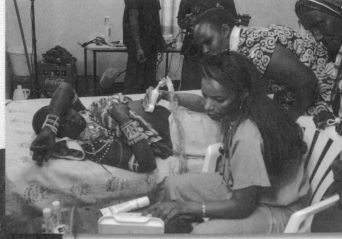

*Working on
behalf
of MFCI*

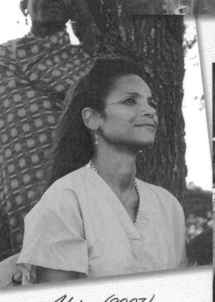

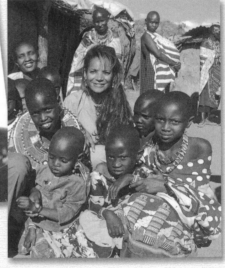

Africa (2007)

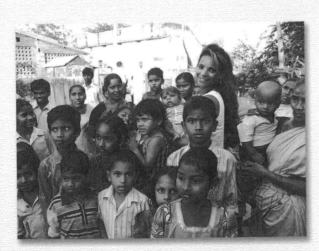

India (2006)

The wonderfully energetic teacher, Paola, introduces us both; then Christophe lets me talk about how FGM affects my life as an ob/gyn and why I am dedicated to helping abolish it. Most of the kids say they haven't heard of the new ban, so Christophe tells them about the law and explains the actual anatomy involved and what really happens during the process.

When we poll them at the beginning, a few kids say they approve of the procedure. I want the whole group to come away from our visit not just saying no to FGM but supportive of changing others. So I spell out the costs. The short-term consequences are dire: death, infection, chronic pain, pain with sex, pain urinating, pain with periods (lots of pain), infertility, the risk of STDs such as hepatitis and HIV/AIDS, which can lead to death. And of course, there are the long-term consequences: dying in labor, dead babies, and obstructed labor leading to the involuntary loss of urine and stool. That last condition, called fistula, leaves women outcast because of their incontinence and infertility.

"Any reason to do this horrible thing to your mother, sister, daughter, or wife?" I ask.

"No!" they say. "No!"

"Let me hear it again!"

"No!" they say, loud and clear.

"Great," I tell them. "I can feel good to go." I feel as though I've turned into a Southern preacher for a moment. But they got it!

I walk back to the hospital nearly exhausted, but I'm hopeful. My patient is there waiting for me. After listening to her history, examining her, and reviewing her previous labs, it's obvious to me that she probably has a bleeding disorder that will require tests that they probably can't do here. I'll have to ask the health director, but it's agonizing that sometimes patients have to go to other countries just to get special lab tests done.

I join my team on labor and delivery and help give the medical students more instruction on ultrasound techniques and fetal heart-rate monitoring. We have a short spaghetti lunch and finish up on the ward, which is quiet now, with only two women in labor. Christophe comes to the hospital and tells me that he got the go-ahead to expand our talks to other schools in Asmara when we return. That means we succeeded today. A step at a time, I tell myself, a step at a time.

Thirty

The Doctors

"No, Richard! I can't take on anything else. Forget it."

I was usually fairly open to the ideas coming at me from my friend and manager Richard Murphy, who'd become an indispensable traffic cop as I fielded requests from TV shows needing experts. But at the end of 2006, all I wanted to think about was the charity—my mind was full of images from Eritrea and Kenya, and I was immersed in planning our next steps.

"You know I wouldn't pull you away from the charity at Christmastime for nothing," Richard said, digging in his heels. "But this is a good one." He'd received a call from a casting director who was interested in me for a medical talk show being put together by the production company behind *Dr. Phil*, and he thought I'd be perfect for it. Fast-talking, energetic, and endlessly enthusiastic, Richard generally thought I'd be perfect for most things, so that by itself wasn't particularly persuasive. But he tended not to push me when he could see my interests were elsewhere. I hated to say no; I just didn't have the energy to pursue this one.

"Lisa, think of the exposure you can get for the charity if you wind up on this show," he said, going for my soft spot.

"Okay, Richard," I answered at last. "Let's say this: You put together the head shot and the background stuff and whatever else they want from me and mail it off. And if something comes of it, I'll follow up."

The rest of the world had slowed to a holiday crawl. There was no way I'd hear from them anytime soon, I thought. But within a week I was driving toward the Paramount Studios lot, where Dr. Phil McGraw and his son Jay McGraw, who'd be the executive producer of the prospective show along with Carla Pennington, would size me up. It was one of the more intimidating meetings I've ever had. Dr. Phil is large in both personality and stature, and at six foot four, he towered over me. I'm five two, and even in heels I felt like a munchkin next to him. But it was easy to answer their questions about me and get in my own queries about the show. By the time we were through, it felt like a real conversation—a good time.

"Brace yourself," Richard said when he called after following up. "They're really interested."

I got a call in January saying, "We definitely want you to be involved," and shortly after that I met the two other doctors who'd been chosen for the show. Travis Stork, an ER doctor from Tennessee who was dynamic enough to star on a season of *The Bachelor,* was stunning on first meeting, tall with the sort of chiseled features that always get my attention. And Drew Ordon, a Beverly Hills plastic surgeon, was a distinguished, good-looking guy with an easy laugh. Jay McGraw invited us to meet at the Polo Lounge at the Beverly Hills Hotel so he could see our chemistry as we got to know each other for the first time. It seems we passed the test, connecting easily and genuinely enjoying one another's company.

For most of the next year we went through a long, slow process of road-testing the concept for the show—they were calling it *The Doctors*—to iron out any kinks. The plan was to have Travis, Drew, and me, and perhaps another doctor or two, talk about the medical news of the day, answer questions from an audience, maybe discuss cases or even perform procedures. For the trial run we'd be recurring guests on Dr. Phil's show.

We struggled with the first segments. The producers wanted us each to be personalities in our own right, but Dr. Phil is such a huge presence himself that I found it hard to shine while I was struggling to adjust to being on stage with someone I admired so much. But we saw from the beginning that we all worked well together, and when we added a fourth doctor, Jim Sears, a genial pediatrician, our group melded.

Before and after every segment we did that year, we'd sit in Dr. Phil's conference room and listen to the producers' feedback about things they'd like us to tweak. Each meeting was like an interview for a job that you'd really like to get, complete with the butterflies of anticipation and the stress of trying to please.

With four people on a stage addressing the same issue, it takes work to strike a balance among them. Finally, though, we developed a natural give-and-take, along with a sweet chemistry. In October I got a call from Jay telling me that we were graduating from *Dr. Phil* to *The Doctors*. "The show's been picked up, and you're on it!" he told me. I was pushing a shopping cart in San Vincente Market and yelled "Yay!" And then I picked up the rest of my groceries. It was Halloween—and I was still Daniel's mom, making chili.

Any ease I'd gained in those practice rounds would be tested as we moved closer to the show's debut in August. Now there was publicity to do, photos to take, a new set and format to master. I thought I'd learned enough over the years to have an easy time of it, but the first year of the show was the challenge of a lifetime, all playing out, of course, on national TV. Friends thought it was fun to see my face on billboards and joked about knowing a "star," but I felt like anything but. I knew the medical information we gave on the show would reach millions of people, and I could feel the weight of the responsibility to get it right and to make full use of the opportunity we had to encourage people to lead healthier lives. And there was so much else to think about. Given my experience at Cedars, I was concerned about how I might be addressed on the show. If the past was any indication, I thought it was quite likely that the guys would be called "doctor" and I'd once again be simply "Lisa." So I was delighted when everyone embraced the easy middle-ground solution: Dr. plus our first names, respect plus a sort of casual, accessible tone. It worked for me—Dr. Travis, Dr. Drew, Dr. Jim, Dr. Lisa.

There seemed to be hundreds of people to meet, and because I'm terrible with names and not great with faces, I was certain they'd write me off as aloof, especially when the day started at seven a.m., an hour I'd always done my best to experience in bed. Worse, I thought they'd find me incompetent. Though I was no newcomer to TV, camera skills alone took a while to master. The set includes a long table where we sit to discuss topics, and the natural thing to do, as the conversation flows, is to turn your head to look at the person speaking. But that drove the cameraman crazy. Apparently, I looked like I was watching a tennis match. Swinging the camera to follow my face every time it turned would be dizzying to viewers, so I had to learn to speak to the camera, or to the audience, instead of the doctor at my side. It's one of those basics I hadn't had occasion to pick up before, and it's a reflex now, but unlearning the habits of a lifetime didn't come easily.

Beyond such logistics we also had volumes of medical content to master. We were taping the show on Thursdays and Fridays, and to prepare we'd each receive a fat white binder on Wednesday evening around five that walked us, segment by segment, through the material we'd be covering. In the beginning we'd just shoot two shows in a day, but as time went on we were asked to do three—and then four—one-hour shows in one long session. Because this was a show about medicine, and my cohosts and I were actually doctors, everyone associated with the show felt a professional responsibility to present the best, most accurate information available. And with an encyclopedia's worth of topics—from swine flu to heart health, nutrition, fitness, cutting-edge treatments, and the ever-popular "most embarrassing bodily functions"—it was a given that we'd want to check and double-check the material, especially when it fell into our specialties.

The producers are experts at what they do, and they made sure we had material in advance so we could help ensure that anything presented on the show was absolutely correct, relying on our expertise as doctors as a final filter. Sometimes I'd make calls to consult with friends in a given specialty to be sure we had the right spin on a new procedure, and I'd check studies myself online if I had questions. I sat with my binder until midnight or later, making notes about what points seemed the most important to stress, and sometimes I'd need to e-mail a segment producer to say, "You know, there's more we need to address here." That's not anyone's preferred activity at eleven the night before an early shoot, but it was better to catch things then than notice a problematic (and unusable) graphic the next morning.

I know I shouldn't have been, but I was truly surprised by the amount of energy the show required. On taping days we'd go through hair and makeup and a morning meeting to discuss the logistics of the different segments and get acquainted with the guests, who range from celebrities (Sally Field! Dr. Ruth! Joan Rivers!) to visiting doctors, and then we'd rush out to shoot the first show, which might, beyond just talking, involve trying out a new fitness routine or demonstrating a procedure or talking a patient through a serious condition. As soon as that show wrapped, we'd duck backstage for a quick wardrobe change and a hair and makeup check, then go out and do it again. I felt like a high school kid, longing for lunch by the end of the second show. We might actually get to eat then, if no one pulled us away for radio interviews. And then: two more shows.

We'd shoot again Friday, and by the end of the day, I was flattened in a way I hadn't been since County. But I also had the same exhilarating sense of satisfaction that I'd felt when I delivered a healthy baby. We were finding a new approach to public health, offering up solid information in a format that was fun to watch. It drew people in. And as the only woman doctor among the hosts, I felt I had a remarkable opportunity to develop a relationship with the female viewers in our audience. It's humbling, and a great honor, to think we can make a difference in people's lives—and like everyone else involved with the show, I felt intense pressure to shine.

I got through the rough early days with the support and hard work of our production team, which patiently taught me what I needed to know. And there was tremendous power in staying connected to the show's mission, which is larger than all of us. In particular I welcomed the chance *The Doctors* afforded to talk about women's health and to empower women, letting them have a voice through me and my cohosts. When the hours got long, and details seemed to swim in my head, I'd tell myself: I'm a Bishop's girl, a County girl, a Mount Holyoke girl, and Baby Rae's girl. What can anyone throw at me that I cannot face? Mom's voice from my middle-school days came through, too. The "be dignified, not jive-y" voice. The one that reminded me that, for the little black girls who just might be watching, I'm a real-life example of the doctor they might one day become.

The show felt like a full-time job, but I had my practice and the rest of my life. I scaled back to two days a week in the office, plus deliveries and emergencies on the days we weren't shooting. And there was still MFCI to run. I've been grateful to be able to travel for the charity for special segments of the show that have taken me back to Kenya and to Sierra Leone, talking about—and showing—the importance of saving the lives of moms and babies there. Erica McGraw, the beautiful young mom who's married to our executive producer Jay McGraw, rolled up her sleeves and joined me on that mission to Kenya, lending her voice and hands to our ongoing work, and my cohosts have participated in fund-raising events. Because of the importance of our work with MFCI, we were also grateful for the support of people like Angela Bassett, Craig Ferguson, and his wife, Megan, connections we could have only dreamed about in our early years. I counted my blessings and kept making phone calls to ask for money and supplies.

At home things were bittersweet. The first year of the show coincided with Daniel's last year of high school, which was packed with activities. I tried to catch as many cello recitals as I could, and on Mondays I still drove him to karate in Hermosa Beach, which could take an hour each way. Sometimes he'd sleep, exhausted from the school day, but often we'd talk and listen to music, just as Mom and I had so many years before. By the time his lesson was over and we'd picked up dinner, it was eight-thirty or nine, almost Tuesday again, and I could feel the show looming.

There were still colleges to check out, campuses to visit, and that big decision hanging over us about where he'd go. Most of the parents of seniors I knew were low-key frantic about helping their kids make the transition to college. I was, too. After all, I was the poster girl for what can happen to smart kids on their own for the first time. Steve was pushing for Amherst, his alma mater, but Daniel had USC in mind, and I couldn't complain. He'd be gone but still within reach.

Early in the run of the show, I could only marvel at the way the pieces of my life had come together. All of us on *The Doctors* got an invitation to a party at the Beverly Hills Hotel to celebrate Dr. Phil's thousandth show, and I couldn't stop smiling when I walked in. "Daniel's going to USC, I just got a TV show, and I'm at a Dr. Phil party," I kept thinking. It was like winning the lottery.

But it was difficult, too. Steve was distant that evening, and from across the room I could see a familiar look in his eyes, the one that said, "I don't see where I fit in." Both our careers had moved just the way we dreamed they would, but in the process we'd come undone. The busier we both became, the harder it was for us to connect. We'd become that couple that talks about the weather and the kid but not each other. That night I was floating with excitement, and when someone came by to whisk me away and introduce me to some of the beautiful people in that beautiful room, Steve retreated to the bar and smoldered. We fought in the car on the way home, replaying a familiar matchup. In one corner: "Why can't you be happy for me?" And in the other corner: "I feel invisible. Is there room for me in your life anymore?"

We went to bed exhausted by the questions that wouldn't go away. Both of us had stopped being able to remember the way we used to relax and enjoy each other's company. And when we got up the next morning, I think we both wondered if we'd lost that ease for good. We were too busy for trauma right then, too busy for endings. But we were unraveling, and pretending couldn't change that. "Mom," I said tearfully to the only person I knew who would understand, "I think it's over."

Thirty-one

Blessings

Work wore me out, but it sustained me, too. The surprise of the first season of *The Doctors* was hearing our name announced as a nominee for a Daytime Emmy® award. And it was sweet confirmation when it happened again the second season. By then I'd settled into a smooth groove, and the other cohosts and I had gotten to know one another not just as doctors but as friends when we'd traveled to Haiti to volunteer our skills after the earthquake in January of 2010. Working side by side in surgery, and seeing patients in the midst of the devastation, I think we gained an even greater respect and affection for each other.

What's made me the happiest are the signs I've gotten that girls are getting the same message from me that I picked up from Diahann Carroll as a kid watching *Julia*: You can do what I do. I was in the airport in Paris when a little girl who told me she was from Saudi Arabia walked up to me and said, "I want to be a doctor, just like you."

I knelt to her level and looked into her eyes. "Thank you," I told her. "I want you to be whatever you want to be, to the best of your ability. If you want to be a doctor, be a doctor. I want you to be what's best for you."

The same thing happened as I waited in the airport on the way to our second Daytime Emmys. A young woman approached me excitedly and said in a rush, "Dr. Lisa! I want to be a doctor, too!

I watch you every day, and I just finished interviewing for med school at UCLA. I don't know how I did in my interviews, but cross your fingers for me."

"If you want to do it," I told her, "keep at it. You'll make it."

"I'll be the first doctor in my family," she said with a smile.

"You're looking at another one right here," I said. "You can do it."

Encounters like that are deeply satisfying to me. I've had a lot of great role models in my life, and if I can give girls a fraction of what I've been given by the women who showed me how to be what I am, I'll feel I've somehow repaid a debt. You have to see an example of what you want before you can reach for it. And the more examples that young black girls—or any girls—can see of a dream that they thought was out of reach, the more possible their dreams become. Yes, I want to tell them, be a doctor. Yes, make a paper dollhouse if paper is all you have, and then make a clinic or a company or your own beautiful life. Yes, take a chance on a wild idea. Yes, give your skills to the people who need them most. Yes, I believe in you.

Proud as we were of our work, and much as we wanted recognition for the producers and the show, I don't think any of us wanted to jinx things by getting overconfident about our Emmy chances. The ceremony was in Las Vegas, and mostly I looked at it as an occasion to spend time with Daniel. I was craving his company and the kind of excitement that I knew he would bring. He and I were in full celebration mode. He'd gone to a concert the night before and hadn't gotten home until morning, so he slept all the way to Vegas. But once we arrived, he walked around the gift suite with me—yes, the gift basket is alive and well—and then played DJ in my room before we went out to dinner with the other docs and their dates, along with our co-executive producer Andrew Scher. Our theme song, "Magic," by B.O.B, made us both feel as though we were in full possession of some stardust of our own.

The morning of the show, Daniel caught me up on his girlfriend and school over breakfast, and later, as I dressed for the show, he helped me practice my teleprompter bits and offered some advice on shoes. He couldn't join me on the red carpet, but I think he gets a kick out of seeing his mom there.

The boys and I would be on early, presenting an award at the beginning of the program, and though the strap came off my shoe as we headed backstage, a magical repair by unseen hands had me ready to go on cue. I think all of us were nervous—not about winning but about being included at the event. It felt as though we'd arrived.

The nerves were gone when we got back to our seats. Against *Dr. Oz* and *Dr. Phil*, I knew the competition was stiff, and everyone from the show seemed relaxed when our category came up. Instead of a short, sweet announcement of the nominees, we were treated to a more "performance art" rendition by Blue Man Group that involved three very blue heads stuck into TV frames, along with some jokey projections and chatter from Alex Trebck. It was all so distracting that it didn't quite register when the logo for *The Doctors* appeared on the Blue Man screens as the winner was announced.

Suddenly, Daniel was yelling, "Mom, Mom, you won! Get up! You won!" Then we were all on our feet, headed for the stage. All I could feel was sheer happiness, and I realized I hadn't been that happy in a long time. Happy for the producers who'd dreamed up the show and made it happen, happy for Travis and Drew and Jim, happy for those poor segment producers who'd taken my calls late at night, happy for all of us who'd created something tangible and good from what had only existed as an idea just a couple of years

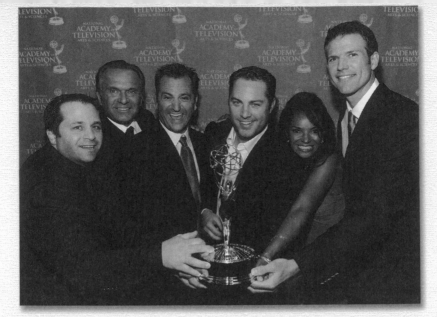

Andrew Scher, Dr. Andrew Ordon, Dr. Jim Sears, Jay McGraw, me, and Dr. Travis Stork after the show's win on Emmy® Night, June 29th, 2010. Photo credit: Frazer Harrison, Getty Images.

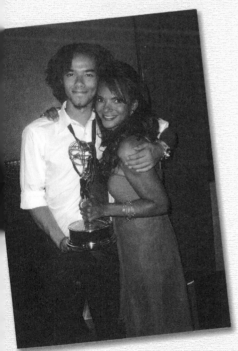

Celebrating with Daniel

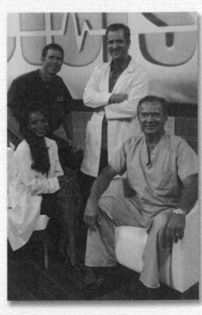

With my co-hosts, Dr. Travis Stork, Dr. Jim Sears, and Dr. Andrew Ordon on the set of The Doctors

Photo credit: Stage 29 Productions and CBS Television Distribution.

before. It's so easy to tune out the acceptance speeches at awards shows, but for once I knew how much they can mean, and I was moved to hear Jay McGraw acknowledge Carla Pennington and Andrew Scher. His parents, Dr. Phil and Robin McGraw. His wife Erica and their new baby.

In my heart there were just a few more words I wished I could add.

As we got into the limo to go to the after party, I looked to the sky and knew what my speech would be.

"Thank you, Mom," I whispered, reaching up my arms and wishing I could hold her. "This is for you."

I may not have had a real dollhouse or even a traditional home growing up, and mine was definitely not a *Leave it to Beaver* family. But I was richly blessed. I had heroes—a mom, a grandma and grandpa, a son and a husband, friends and mentors—who taught me to believe in myself and who showed me the power of connecting with a mission that was larger than just me.

They were and are real people, perfect in their very human imperfection. My life's been all about finding the gift in the imperfections, learning by doing, failing, and getting up again. It's not a straight, smooth path, but it's been an amazing one.

There's so much yet to do. We're still in negotiations with tribal leaders over land for a larger clinic in Kenya. I've seen unfathomable need in Sierra Leone and Kenya and India and Eritrea.

The trip I took to Sierra Leone for *The Doctors*, in particular, gave me a sense of urgency about what groups like MFCI—and all of us—must find a way to do. I'd read an article in the *Los Angeles Times* in late 2009 that made me curious about how we might help in that country, which is in the same region of Africa as Ghana.

Sierra Leone is still recovering from a decade of civil war between 1991 and 2001, and the impact of the country's political turmoil on women and children has been acute. Of every one thousand babies born there, one hundred and twenty-three die. Those who survive have a life expectancy of just forty-eight years (up from forty during the war). And over a lifetime a woman there has a one in eight chance of dying in childbirth.

Our visit to Freetown, the country's capital, was greeted with great excitement, and First Lady Sia Koroma, a psychiatric nurse who has devoted herself to helping solve the country's health-care crisis, met us when we arrived. She spent a day introducing us to government health officials and showing us around a clinic. It was a sobering sight. The hospital had no running water, and the high-risk pregnancy ward was bluntly referred to as the death ward. Every basic you can imagine was in short supply or missing. In a city of shelled buildings that still need repair, it's not just a matter of bringing ambulances and sutures. First, there must be roads, shelter, safe drinking water.

Mrs. Koroma asked if we could build birthing clinics in rural areas, as we had in Kenya. And we can, if we find new ways to spread empathy, information, and resources. Challenges like this exist around the world, and working together, we can take them on—and make life better. MFCI will be raising funds and partnering with other organizations to help make that happen. I hope you will find ways, large or small, to help.

The UN Millennium Development Goals for reducing mortality rates of pregnant women and babies around the world still daunt us. And girls everywhere need support to be as smart and brave and self-reliant as they can be. I was recently asked to be a spokesperson for a new UN Foundation program called Girl Up, which encourages young women to give a "High Five"—a donation of five dollars or more—to help their peers in developing countries. Girls can learn early to help each other, supporting programs that provide education, health care, clean water, and more. As a Champion for Girl Up, I'll be traveling to see and talk about the impact of those efforts.

Whatever your age, you can make a difference. Don't forget to try. Whatever it is you dream of, take a step toward it. Then take one more. Let me inspire you, and let your actions inspire someone else. The world needs all of us to be our own heroes.

My mom died at fifty-three, and though my health is great and I can see the good genes of others in my family, I still feel the same sense of urgency I've had all my life. To squeeze in more, keep going, make one more phone call, say yes to that last bit of "extra credit," hold my son a little longer as he steps out into the world. To try to save another baby.

I haven't yet learned to stop moving, and I haven't spun fast enough to turn into Wonder Woman, either. But somehow I think my mom believes I can do both someday. I have a feeling that she's with me still, whispering, "We'll find a way."

Acknowledgments

This book would not have been possible without the
love, support, and patience of the following people:

My wonderful staff at Ocean Oasis, Linda Buttles, Patty Villa, Karin Johnston.

All of the producers, crew, and production staff on *The Doctors*.

My patients, who inspire me and make me appreciate being a doctor every day.

The doctors and donors who continue to support
Maternal Fetal Care International.

Donna Lane, my MFCI champion.

My teachers at Epiphany, Bishop's, Mount Holyoke,
USC Medical School and their residency program.

The best teachers in my life, my mother and grandmother.

Stephen and Daniel Masterson.

My Uncle Don, Uncle Almer, and my brother, Christopher.

Richard G. Murphy, Janice Goldklang, Marc Golden, Esq., BJ Robbins,

and especially Donna Frazier Glynn.